GOOD PO

Erika Lust

Translated by X. P. Callahan

Good Porn
A Woman's Guide

Published by
Seal Press
A Member of the Perseus Books Group
1700 Fourth Street
Berkeley, California

Library of Congress Cataloging-in-Publication Data

Lust, Erika.
  [Porno para mujeres. English]
  Good porn : a woman's guide / Erika Lust ; translated by X. P. Callahan.
       p. cm.
  Includes bibliographical references.
  ISBN 978-1-58005-306-8
 1. Pornographic films--History and criticism. 2. Women and erotica.
I. Title.
  PN1995.9.S45L86813 2010
  791.43'6538--dc22

2009053793

10 9 8 7 6 5 4 3 2 1

Cover design by Silverander Communications
Interior design by Tabitha Lahr
Printed in the United States of America
Distributed by Publishers Group West

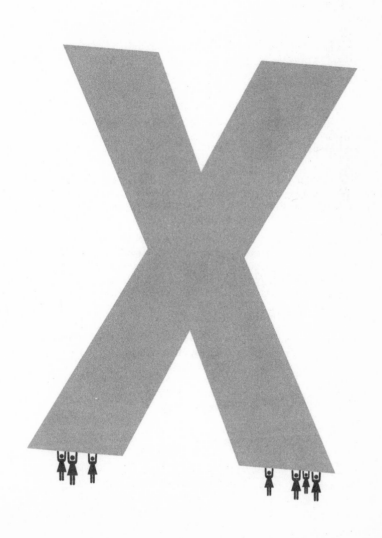

CONTENTS

1. Porn for Men-----13
On the clichés of porn producers and directors (no, women don't really wear spike heels in bed) and their movies' awful sets, music, costumes, and actors.

2. Women, Feminism, and Pornography-----25
Why watch porn? Because we have the same right as men to get ourselves off. Forget flowers, cozy fires, and romance—we want porn where we call the shots.

3. The History of Porn-----43
Hic habitat felicitas—two thousand years of sex, from the murals of Pompeii to the Internet.

4. FAQs-----59
"How do pornographic movies get made?" "Are the women in porn abused?" "Does that position really exist?" "My boyfriend's isn't *that* big!" Everything you ever wanted to know about pornographic films—but were afraid to ask.

5. A Dictionary of Porn-----71
Rim job, money shot, CFNM, English discipline, blow job, golden shower, gang bang, facial, R-18, *kokigami*, MET Art—learn the arcane language of pornographic films so you can find what you want, without making yourself sick.

6. Horror Movies, Comedies, and Porn-----81
Horror movies should give you chills, comedies should make you laugh, and porn should make you hot. Learn how to find what really turns you on.

PREFACE

In the beginning, porn struck me the same way it strikes most women. It was anything but love at first sight. Obviously, there was something about the images that turned me on, but there were also a lot of things that bothered me.

I couldn't see myself in those films—not my lifestyle or my values, and not my sexuality. They didn't portray female pleasure at all, and the women in those movies existed for one reason alone—to pleasure the men. The sexual situations were ridiculous, too, based on male fantasies. (For example, a girl comes home and catches her guy in bed with her best friend, but instead of getting mad, she decides to hop in and join the party.)

Not only that, people my age had grown up with MTV, so we found adult films' production values totally unacceptable. The cheesy sets, the awful styling and makeup, the insipid music, the laughable performances (with sound editing that was even worse), and the amateurish cinematography—it all made for a very inferior product.

And the men making adult films back then expected their audiences to put up with female stereotypes that had already been offending modern women for a good twenty years. I soon had my fill of horny Lolitas, kinky teenagers, fuck bunnies constantly in the mood, desperate women, hot nurses, nympho hookers, and semen-slugging heroines. Women like these may have represented the feminine sexual ideal for guys, but they left me cold. Then there were the male characters—almost all of them were Mafia dons, pimps, drug lords, arms dealers, bazillionaires, or sickly muscled sex machines hung like a horse. For guys, maybe, these men were sexual heroes, but they didn't do a thing for me.

So I had my criticisms of the adult film genre, as you can see. But even though I didn't like what I was seeing, something inside me was pushing me to look deeper. I discovered that there were quite a few feminist intellectuals who also hated porn, but they hadn't stopped there. They had gone on to analyze it as a contemporary cultural phenomenon. Two books by Linda Williams, *Hard Core* and *Porn Studies*, inspired me. After reading them, I decided to become a porn producer and director myself. I understood that a different kind of porn was possible, and that women had a great deal to contribute to a genre that had always been the exclusive province of men.

Today there are a lot of us out there—women who like watching well-made films that include sexually explicit content, even though we've so often been disappointed by efforts to make such films. But some of us have kept our eyes open while swimming against the tide, and we've become what we might call "wise wankers"—women who know what we want, and what we don't.

In this book, I want to be your guide to the intricate world of adult films. Together we'll discover how to take some chances with this controversial genre, and how to approach it without losing our feminine critical eye. We have to be able to enjoy ourselves without feeling insulted.

Have fun!

Erika Lust
Barcelona, Spain

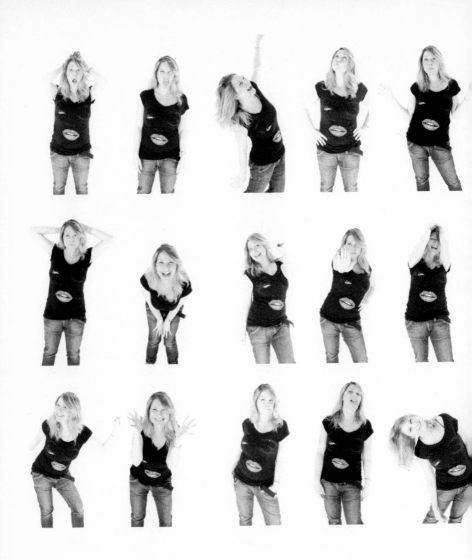

ENJOY!

WOMEN'S VOICES

Eliza

It blows my mind how awful the music in porn films is! Lots of times I just turn the volume all the way down and put my own sound track on. And they take two hours to tell these completely ridiculous stories—I can't stand it. But the worst are the remakes—*Gladiator X, Mission Possible, Charlie's Sex Angels*. Instead of making you horny, they just crack you up.

Violet Blue (www.tinynibbles.com)

Mostly, porn should be fun, hot, wankable. But I think it can be pretty liberating, too. Set yourself up to challenge anti-porn pundits and sex-negative points of view by becoming a clever consumer armed with self-knowledge about porn's positive effects on your own sex life. We need to break down cultural myths about porn's degradation of women and its mythical ability to cause rape and child molestation, and to create "porn addicts."

Angelica

Why are the guys in pornographic movies such fat, short, ignorant assholes? And they're always pushing themselves on pretty girls! It's not like that in real life. But if the point is to tell lies, then why can't we see plain Janes hooking up with hot guys, or much younger boys? Take any pornographic movie, and the casting will reek of male chauvinism.

Candida Royalle (www.candidaroyalle.com)

It seemed to me that most porn was sex-negative and did not present a woman's point of view or show what women liked sexually. At the same time I could tell women were becoming more curious and felt permission to explore their sexuality. . . . I saw a challenging new market.

Karina

Lots of my women friends give me a hard time because I'm always saying how much I adore the blonde bombshells in American porn—those tall, curvy chicks with their tigress fingernails. I don't know why, but they turn me on. Probably because there aren't any women like that around here, or because those women are like a cartoon version of sexuality. A good example is Jenna Jameson before she turned anorexic. What I don't like, though, is how they're dressed and made up to look like whores. I'd rather see them in jeans and a T-shirt, wearing Converse sneakers instead of six-inch spike heels.

Tristan Taormino (www.puckerup.com)

Porn has always been, and continues to be, a huge issue for women. I don't know if the debate will ever be over. But it's hard to hear from other feminists. They haven't seen my porn, they haven't seen Candida Royalle or Belladonna. So they don't see that porn is not one monolithic thing that's all bad.

Anna

I want real plots, believable characters, and ordinary people I can identify with. In most of these movies, the guys are Mafia kingpins, drug dealers, multimillionaires, prison guards . . . tough guys who treat girls like sex toys. I never see myself! I want to see real men, men like my friends, men who treat women like equals, with love and respect.

Rebecca

Porn is like a guy who's a libertine, but sexist and conservative. He doesn't mind asking you and another woman to put on a show for him, but if you so much as suggest that he let another man touch him, he's shocked, as if you'd asked him to kill somebody.

Erika Lust (www.erikalust.com)

I belong to a generation whose modern, diverse sexuality is not represented in traditional male-oriented pornography. We women need to take steps now to start changing the views of sex that men have been putting out there through porn. If we don't, then future generations won't have anything but that diminished, impoverished vision of sexuality.

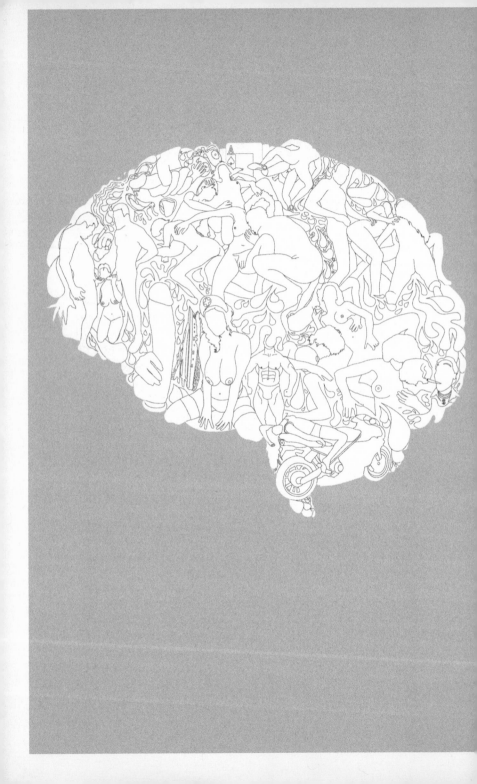

CHAPTER 1
PORN FOR MEN

AN OPEN LETTER TO THE MEN WHO PRODUCE AND DIRECT PORNOGRAPHIC FILMS

Gentlemen:

The time has come to admit what we all know. For decades you've had a monopoly on defining what porn is, and you've been making adult films that express your own ideas, desires, and fantasies. The porn that now infests the world represents your sexuality and yours alone.

But the time has come for you to open your private, secret world to women. In politics, we've already managed to crash the party. Now we want access to *your* private preserve, and as soon as we get in, we're going to want some changes. Because we are not happy. We are not satisfied.

When I decided to start making erotic and sexually explicit films especially for women, you guys in the industry accused me of being outmoded and backward. You told me it was discriminatory to make films just for women. You said you were already making movies that were for everyone.

But that's not true. Your films are male-oriented, and in this world of ours, whatever is male-oriented becomes the standard, so it never occurred to you that something might be missing. You thought everybody on the planet liked what you like. It's the same as when a school holds a parents' night, but the only parents who show up are mothers, or when only the word "mankind" is used to talk about humanity as a whole.

These days, women directors are popping up all over the world. When we talk about making films for women, it's not because we want to exclude men from our audiences. We're just pointing out that our movies are made with a female audience in mind, and that the focus of our movies is female pleasure and desire—which basically proves that your own films aren't primarily intended for women.

So what are you afraid of? Instead of circling the wagons and trying to keep us out, why not take a look at our films? If you watch our movies, maybe you'll understand how we see things. Maybe you'll even like them, the same way many of us like male-oriented porn.

Wouldn't it be great if we really had free choice and could take our pick of female- or male-oriented films? These days we can go to a newsstand and buy male- or female-oriented magazines, whether we're men or women, and whether we're gay, lesbian, or transgender. But when it comes to pornographic films, the only ones we can get are yours, and yours are one-dimensional and all the same.

Lucía Etxebarría is one of my favorite Spanish writers, and her latest book is an anthology that she edited. It's called *If Men Only Knew . . . Women Talk About Sex*. Here's what she has to say in her magnificent preface: "It's no accident that in commercial sex films intended for male audiences—that is, porn—women are almost always portrayed as things, as victims. The camera may linger fondly over the man's ejaculation, but the same attention is rarely paid to the woman's sexual enjoyment." She goes on to say that "pornographic films in general are produced and directed by men and intended for male audiences, so they're tightly focused on a

14

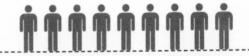

handful of highly specific codes—objectifying and humiliating women, and always keeping male pleasure front and center."[1]

Etxebarría is right, and what she's saying is something I discovered for myself. At one time, way back before I even thought about starting Lust Films, I was doing audiovisual production work for advertising and films, including pornographic films. One big distribution and production company where I worked wanted to launch a new line for women, or at least that's what they said. But they had the bright idea of putting a man in charge of it, and of course the project was a huge flop. That was my first contact with the porn industry, and I quickly realized that this was a world controlled by men who were not really all that professional. I also realized that I had quite a lot to say, and quite a lot to give, to young people today, and especially to other women.

But the problem is not just that the porn industry is controlled by men. It's the *kind* of men they are. To be specific, these men are unhip, anti-feminist, anti-intellectual, and unenlightened. There are exceptions, obviously, but most of these men are pretty dumb. And they're all pretty much alike. As I got to know the men in the adult film business, I came to understand why their movies are so indistinguishable. There's no racial or sociocultural diversity among these producers and directors. And because they're all alike, they all think alike. They're mostly middle-aged straight white guys, and their taste in women runs to big-breasted horny blonde airheads. It just stands to reason that a homogenous group is going to create a homogenous product.

I've actually seen screenplays less than three pages long for porn films that lasted an hour. The writers used maybe six words for the typical scene:

"BLONDE fucks BLACK GUY in KITCHEN." And for the rest of the scenes, they just substituted different words for the words in caps.

The men who make traditional pornographic films think that set decoration is all about ancient Rome and spaceships, and that locations are about shooting in some palatial house on the Costa Azul or in the Seychelles. That's how they make a new movie look different from the one that came before. As far as I'm concerned, though, this is just a bunch of boring male fantasy, or maybe it's nothing but an excuse for the producers and directors to travel. But we women can just have our film shoots in a loft, or on a bed. We're not trying to impress anybody with our luxury cars or jet skis. When we want to impress people, we can point to our actors' performances, or our screenplays, or the rhythms of our plots, or the quality of the sex.

The new films that women are making for women are all about intimacy and relationships. The films that men make are about ass fucking and ejaculations. From the very beginnings of the porn industry, men have had a stranglehold on how we define porn and how we think about it. But it's our turn now, mine and other women's, to redefine what porn can and must be—for *us*.

Films obviously made by men, with men in mind

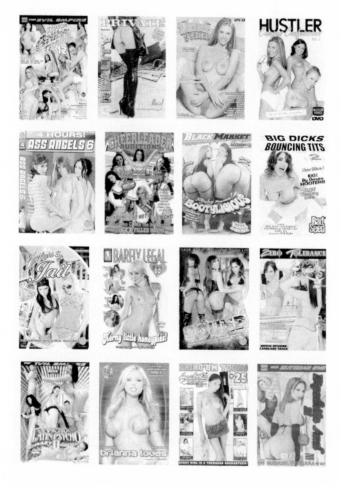

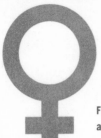

Films with more appeal to women, made with different values and a different aesthetic

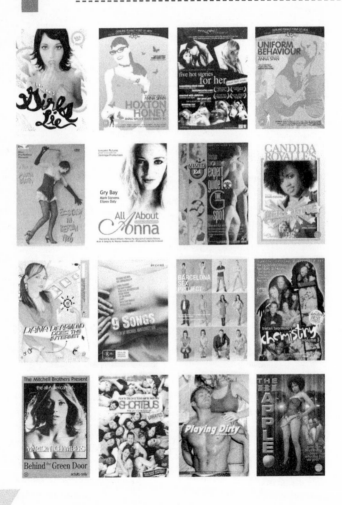

♂ IN PORN FOR MEN . . .   ♀ IN PORN FOR WOMEN . . .

Oral Sex	
Deep Throat-style blow jobs	Cunnilingus

Setting	
A luxurious mansion	A modern apartment

Male Characters	
Mafia kingpins, drug dealers, spies, soldiers, jailers	Typical guys like the ones you know

Female Characters	
Blonde hookers, nymphomaniacs, lesbians who fuck guys, secret agents/hired killers, kinky teenagers	Typical modern women who have jobs and are sexually liberated—women like you and your friends

Technology and Transportation	
Sports cars, jet skis, helicopters, private jets	iPhones, Macs, Minis, Vespas

Beliefs and Attitudes	
Girls are always in the mood; deep down, women enjoy rape	Sex has to be earned (she doesn't spread her legs just because he asks her to), and it has to be consensual

Women's Costumes	
Net stockings; a miniskirt fit for a hooker; a skimpy top; ridiculous high heels or platform shoes	A sexy Miss Sixty, Armani, or Mango dress; jeans and a T-shirt

19

STRANGE BUT TRUE

It's not just the adult film business that shuts women out. We're noticeably scarce in the audiovisual industry as a whole. Only one woman has won an Oscar for best director (Kathryn Bigelow, 2010), and only four women have ever been nominated—not because women's movies aren't good enough, but because almost no women are making movies. We don't get the high-level jobs in the industry, so we don't get the same opportunities men enjoy. For more of this kind of information, check out the Guerrilla Girls (www.guerillagirls.com). (At least in the future billboards like the one featured below will be able to claim a single female win for Best Director!)

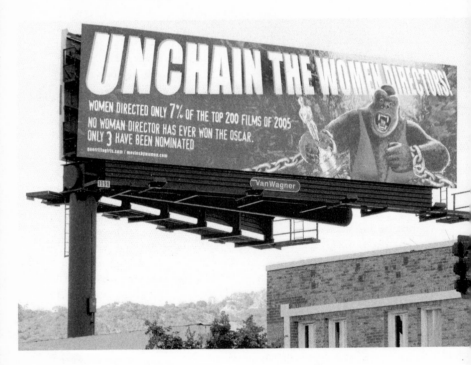

IN THE PHONY, PREDICTABLE PORN MADE BY MEN . . .

1. Women wear spike heels to bed.

2. Men can always get it up.

3. When a man goes down on a woman, ten seconds is more than enough for her.

4. If a woman is masturbating and a man she doesn't know walks in on her, she's never afraid or embarrassed. She just invites him to have sex with her.

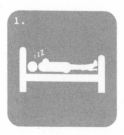  

5. Men always shoot a pint or more.

6. When a man is choking a woman with his dick, she always smiles and enjoys it.

7. Beautiful young women just love to have sex with fat, ugly, middle-aged men.

8. Men and women always come at the exact same instant.

9. A blow job can fix a traffic ticket or settle any kind of debt.

10. Every woman screams like a banshee when she comes.

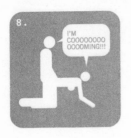  

11. All women have big beautiful boobs, and all men have big beautiful cocks.

12. Double penetration feels good to a woman and makes her beam with delight.

13. Asian men do not exist.

14. Men with small dicks also do not exist.

15. If you should run across a couple fucking in a park or in the woods, go ahead and shove your dick into the girl's mouth—the guy won't beat

 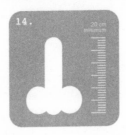 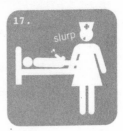

the crap out of you.

16. Every woman loves to get fucked in the ass.

17. Nurses always suck their patients' cocks.

18. Men always pull out before they come.

19. If your wife or girlfriend discovers you in

bed with her best friend, she'll be mad for a second or two, but then she'll decide to make it a threesome.

20. A woman never has a headache, and she never gets her period.

21. Women enjoy dressing up like whores or little girls.

22. When a woman is sucking a man's cock, it's important for him to give her constant reminders about what to do: "Oh yeah—suck it!"

23. Butts are always squeaky-clean and tasty, and a woman loves to pull a dick out of her butt and pop it right into her mouth.

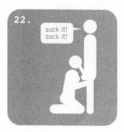  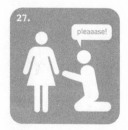

24. A woman is always pleasantly surprised when she unzips a man's pants and discovers a dick in there.

25. Even when she's being raped, a woman always shouts, "Yes! Yes! Harder!" Every woman secretly wants to be raped.

26. Every lesbian is tall, thin, and pretty and has long hair and nails.

27. Men never have to ask, of course, because every woman is always in the mood for a good fuck.

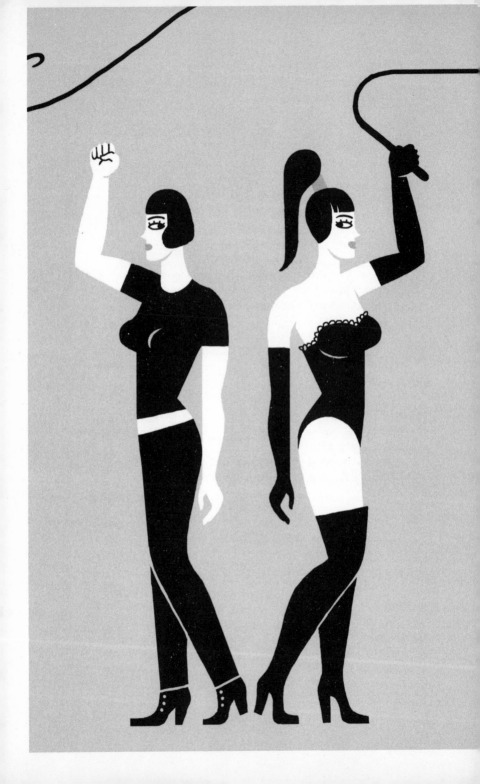

CHAPTER 2
WOMEN, FEMINISM, AND PORNOGRAPHY

QUESTIONS

Should women watch porn?

Adult films seem like a genre that women should hate, one that women have traditionally been expected to hate. But should we challenge that cliché? Can you be a feminist as well as someone who likes porn, or are the two incompatible?

Is porn depraved, or can it help us learn about sexuality?

Does porn turn us into porn addicts, or can it help us have more fun in bed?

Is porn dirty? Does it kill desire, or can it fire up the libido?

Do we need to fight and censor porn, or should we participate in this male-oriented phenomenon to change it and shape it to our own tastes?

ANSWERS

One thing is for sure—as a group, we women haven't had much time to exercise our right to enjoy our bodies and our sexuality. Remember, even today there are cultures that are still using barbaric practices like clitoridectomy to nip female sexual desire in the bud.

Not so long ago, women's sexuality was powerfully conditioned—or repressed—by society, the patriarchy, the church, puritan moralism, and even training in female subservience, which some girls got at home. These institutions, all dominated by men, have spent hundreds of years trying to heap blame on us and fill us with fear so they can keep our sexuality under control, and especially so they can remind us that sex, for women, is closely tied to reproduction and men's sexual pleasure. Remember that even today, in the same social and cultural circles where women are looked down on for having multiple sexual partners, there's nothing but admiration for a man who has multiple partners.

I BELIEVE IN PORN

I believe in porn's potential to help women keep our sexual revolution going. This fight is far from over, so it has to be kept alive. It wasn't settled in the 1970s—it was just getting started.

I believe we can benefit from watching sexually explicit films. We're sexually liberated these days, and we can find pornographic images that will inspire us to follow our bliss. Porn can help us spice up our fantasies and discover tastes we never even knew we had.

And porn can be an instrument of education and liberation for women who are still struggling with shame, guilt, and sexual repression. We can see that desires and fantasies we thought were abnormal are actually quite common. As women, we have to give ourselves permission to explore our sexuality.

> *Not only do we have to learn to enjoy sex, we have to demand our right to sexual pleasure.*

For Kate Millett, "there is some usefulness in explicitness" because it can help women recover from "dreadful patriarchal ideas that sex is evil and that the evil in it is women"; see the interview with Millett by Linda Williams, *Hard Core: Power, Pleasure, and the "Frenzy of the Visible"* (Berkeley: University of California Press, 1999).

> *Some of the women who say they don't like porn have never watched even a single frame of a pornographic movie, so their rejection of porn is traditional and conventional, with no basis in objective reality.*

In the Victorian era, as we'll see in the next chapter, the puritans took care to keep pornography under wraps and make it available only to upper-class men, always behind closed doors in private libraries or all-male clubs. They kept an iron grip on this material because they thought it might arouse uncontrollable desires if it were to fall into the wrong hands—hands weaker than their own. So they tried to shield their "inferiors" from sex in all its depravity. And who were the ones banished from sexuality? Who were these vulnerable beings who couldn't be trusted with sex? They were women, children, and anyone from the lower classes. Only a man of means could be admitted to the secret world of sex.

But the notion of sex as something dirty is fairly recent. It reached full flower with the puritanism of the nineteenth century (graphic representations of sex were not considered obscene in ancient cultures). This repressive attitude had originally taken root at the high point of Judeo-Christian culture, when sex was gradually coming to be seen as forbidden fruit. Recall what the "holy" Bible says—that Eve, that slut, tempted poor innocent Adam with an apple and brought the noble purity of man and all of Paradise to ruin.

With the spread of Judeo-Christian norms and morals all over the West, people began to discriminate between acceptable, pure, noble culture (a culture of chastity, virginity, purity, and Stoicism) and low, dirty, immoral culture (the culture to which representations of sex were consigned). Hedonism became a forbidden philosophy of life.

But in today's world there's no place for that kind of discrimination. Even though so much bad porn is aesthetically and morally ugly, porn in and of itself is not a bad thing.

WHAT DO WOMEN WANT TO SEE?

Let's start by clearing up the number one question people ask me: *Just what is it that women want to see in porn? What do they like? What turns women on?*

The answer? We want to see everything.

What do you mean, everything?

I mean we want to see everything—and nothing!

And here's the typical response: *I don't understand.*

Women want romance—and rough sex. We want sensitive men—and brutes who manhandle us. We want to see genitals—and we'd rather not. We want to see handsome, muscular models—and normal-looking guys. We want violins and true love—and zipless fucks. Our tastes are as varied as men's are.

It's difficult to make sweeping statements about what half the world's population wants. Women can't be pigeonholed into a single monolithic category. This may sound like a validation of the claim we hear from men (and some women)—that we don't need female-oriented adult films—but in fact it's not.

WHAT MODERN WOMEN WANT IN ADULT FILMS

We Are Visual

The first cliché that needs to be challenged is the one that says women don't like looking at sexually explicit images but would rather see suggestive, erotic, softcore pictures showing simulations of sex. Supposedly, most of us are less visually oriented than men are and get less turned on than men do watching representations of sex. But that's a myth. A while ago, I was talking with some *Hustler* executives in Los Angeles, and they acknowledged that women account for 50 percent of sales in their *Hustler* Hollywood megastore on Sunset Boulevard. And websites like Suicide Girls and I Feel Myself and Beautiful Agony have quite a few women subscribers. Obviously, then, we do like looking at pictures of sex. This freaks a lot of men out, but they should get used to the idea that if they can jerk off at their computers or in front of the TV or with a magazine, so can we.

So hold the flowers and fireplaces, the candles and romance novels by Danielle Steele. We want sexually explicit images, but we want to call the shots when it comes to how they're made.

Our Films' Values

We want films that are made for adult women, films that show us real women, films that tell us about our sexuality. We don't want to be portrayed as passive objects or victims but as active subjects giving and receiving pleasure. We want to see other women enjoying themselves.

We don't want to see the typical strong, independent "man of mystery" who's in tune with himself and his feelings and who takes a sensitive, dependent woman—a woman totally out of touch with her body and her sexuality—and helps her discover

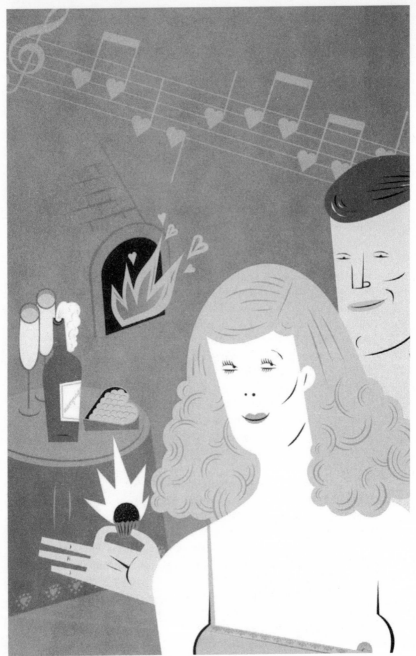

Mythbusting: Women don't always need a romantic atmosphere to have sex a whole world of sensations. The type of man who opens up the world to women—the type of man women would be lost without—is a type that particularly sets my nerves on edge. And what's most annoying is when the actor playing that role also happens to be the film's producer and director. (Believe me, that's been done, and more than once.)

So what kind of men do we want to see? We want to see modern men who share our values, men who respect women, men we find attractive. A man doesn't have to be Prince Charming. Everybody knows that we women can become attached to men we're not initially attracted to, since we can appreciate their other qualities, such as personality and spirit. And every now and then we might even want to see two men together.

I've spent my whole career talking with other women about what we like in a man, and even though it's not really possible to generalize, it's clear that most of us don't lose our heads over the typical porn hero—the macho superstud with a huge dick, like Rocco Siffredi or Nacho Vidal. Those two have climbed to the top of the porn world on the backs of men who aren't as well muscled or as well hung, men who get turned on watching them in tours de force like *Rocco Ravishes Prague* or *Reverse Gang Bang: Twenty Girls for Rocco and Nacho*. But if you've watched any of the gonzo porn by these two male superstars, you've already seen how they push women to the limit. That's generally a turnoff for us, a point I'll make as often as necessary.

But when I say it's generally a turnoff, I'm choosing my words carefully. Some women actually are turned on by the fantasy or experience of violent, aggressive sex. And I'm not saying a good hard fuck bordering on rape can't be interesting from a woman's perspective, but I do think it has to take place with her clear consent.

Linda Williams says something very interesting in her book *Hard Core*. She says that one of the most hackneyed fantasies staged in male porn is the rape that turns into ecstatic sex, with the woman finally coming. Men always imagine that "no" means "yes." Hence the classic problem of rape in our sexist society—the suspicion that the victim was asking for it. That's why our courts have such a hard time with rape, and why victims of rape are often assumed to be lying—if they bother to report the crime at all.

And that's why I *really* don't like it when a girl in a movie is supposedly being raped but keeps shouting, "Yes! Yes! I like that! Harder!" For the most part, *this is nothing but a male fantasy*. "Yes" means "yes," and "no" does mean "no."

We Want to See Ourselves

We don't want to see female characters who exist in the collective male imagination or in the world of men's ideal sexual fantasies—the prostitutes, the baby sitters, the horny teenyboppers, the schoolgirls with pigtails and miniskirts and lollipops, the nymphos, the cheerleaders who blow every guy on the team, the multiorgasmic waitresses, the *Baywatch* babes. No, we've had quite enough of men turning women into whores in their pornographic films. Or let me put it this way—go ahead and keep making the same adult movies; somebody will like them. But modern women like me want to see *ourselves* in a new kind of adult film for women. We want to see a woman restaurateur, a smart woman business executive, a woman president, a single mother, a married mother, a graphic designer, a clerk in a sex toy store. We want to see normal women performing in movies about real sex, movies in which intimacy is front and center, movies in which we can get to know the characters before we see them fucking.

Stills from *Breakup Sex* (www.cincohistorias.com)

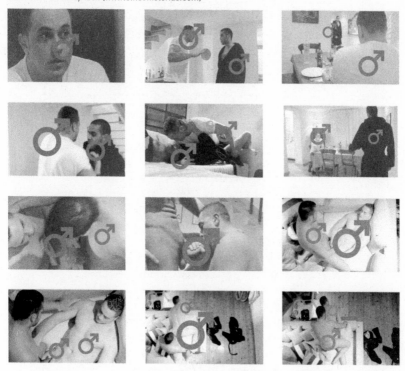

Every pornographic film has a girl-on-girl scene, but when I included a guy-on-guy scene in *Five Hot Stories for Her,* people looked at me like I was crazy. It doesn't bother men at all to be turned on by a lesbian sex scene, but they totally lose it when we want to see sex between two men.

> *Not many women find it inviting to watch some cigar-chomping, brandy-guzzling mafia kingpin give orders to a bunch of muff-diving teenagers who then take turns fucking the old coot.*

When a guy watches porn, he's hoping the actresses will get their clothes off and get down to the business of blowing the male lead, the sooner the better. All he wants from the female characters is tits and ass. He doesn't care about the color or pattern of the sheets, or about set decoration or music or makeup—or he does, but only if they show what sluts the women are in their whorish makeup and platform shoes, at the mansion of whichever millionaire has invited them to share his Jacuzzi.

But I think we women need a new aesthetic for adult films, one that will cover everything from the clothing worn by male and female performers to the design of the DVD box. From time immemorial, the feminine has usually been more stylish and better designed than the masculine, so why shouldn't that also be true when it comes to porn? Ours will just be prettier.

The porn world is changing as sexual minorities call attention to their lack of representation in adult films. Lesbians have been organizing to make realistic, sexually explicit films in which not everyone is a slender blonde beauty with long nails and platform shoes. Transpeople and cross-dressers want to appear onscreen, too—there's a lively market in drag films, and now women who feel themselves to be men are also demanding their place. The gay male community may be the only minority group that has been making its own adult movies for years, creating a solid genre and a large body of work.

So what about straight women? As it happens, we're assumed to be sufficiently represented in the genre of straight male porn, and we're supposed to be satisfied with that. But I'm speaking out against that belief. The heterosexual porn in which we're supposedly represented is actually for straight men. It's made by straight men and intended for straight men. There are no women in the adult entertainment industry, other than actresses, makeup artists, and a few women here and there in low-level positions. And if there are no women producing, writing, or directing adult films, then there won't be any adult films that have our sensibilities and our point of view.

FEMINISM

I'm going to talk now about feminism. Why? Because when I say that I make pornographic feminist films, more than a few people think I'm attempting to mix oil with water. I also believe, like many other feminists, that feminism can and should permeate every corner of cultural and artistic expression, pornography included.

All too often I find myself among men, and women, who simply don't know what feminism is. They usually believe, quite wrongly, that we feminists are an army of unattractive women determined to wipe men off the face of the earth. It really makes me mad to see how many people today still use the word "feminist" as the worst kind of insult. And I continue to feel that in many social settings you're branded as dangerous or a troublemaker if you're a woman who isn't meek and mild, or if you ask too many questions, or if you're demanding or pushy or out of line. So let's take a look at just what this thing called feminism is, or at least I'll explain how I see it.

The conflict that gave rise to feminism has to do with actual differences between men and women. We live in a world in which women and men don't have the same possibilities, rights, and opportunities, a world in which women as a group have less power than men as a group, even though women make up more than 50 percent of the world's population. Being a feminist means acknowledging this situation and believing that it should change.

And how will it change? We need to be specific about what the differences are between men and women before we can move on to the next stage—changing the conditions of inequality. So if you think women are already enjoying the same possibilities, rights, and conditions as men, here are a few facts for you:

♀ In most democracies, let alone nondemocratic societies, there are far more men than women in major political posts.

♀ The world of business and high finance has almost no women at the top.

♀ Men earn more money than women, and different salaries are often paid to men and women who are doing the same work.

♀ If a woman lives with a man and has a job outside the home, and especially if she has children, she actually has two jobs, since women still do most of the housework and child care.

♀ In developing countries, fewer girls than boys go to school, and in some of those countries a female fetus can be aborted just for being female.

I like to say that feminists are antisexist. We all know the negative connotations of sexism, and to be a feminist is to fight the injustices produced by the sexism that still rules our society. It seems to me that being antisexist makes as much sense as being antiracist or antihomophobic.

MACHISMO

Machismo[1] encompasses a set of attitudes, behaviors, social practices, and beliefs intended to rationalize and promote the maintenance of discrimination toward women, and toward men whose behavior is not sufficiently "masculine" in the eyes of those imbued with macho ideology.

Traditionally, machismo has been associated with the hierarchization and subordination of roles within the family so as to enhance the comfort and well-being of men. In this sense, it is a manifestation of machismo to assign men more rewarding or less tiring work without fair and justifiable criteria for doing so. Another aspect of machismo is the use of any type of violence against women if its purpose is to keep women under emotional or hierarchical control. But even when expressions of machismo are psychological rather than physical, it is regarded as a form of coercion because it tends to preserve discrimination, undermining women's abilities with claims that women are the weaker sex. Machismo also forms the basis of homophobia, since it comes down hard on behavior in males that could be seen as feminine.

According to feminists, machismo constitutes oppression of the female sex and is a major social scourge. It also accounts for at least some amount of domestic violence, also known as macho violence.

FEMINISM AND PORN: FELLOW TRAVELERS

Now that we've seen what feminism is, let's look at how it's related to porn. Feminism and porn have always had a love-hate relationship. The feminist movement has traditionally opposed pornography, since porn is clearly and obviously a practice that exploits and assaults women. Such major feminist gurus as Andrea Dworkin and Catharine MacKinnon launched fierce attacks against pornography, using highly persuasive arguments in addition to slogans like "Porn is the theory; violence is the practice."[2]

But that posture has softened over time. Today there are modern, very broad currents of feminism that don't view porn as the enemy. The anticensorship forces have evolved into the sex-positive movement. We consider a woman at liberty to use her body however she pleases, and we're decidedly in favor of sexual freedom. Here is how Wendy McElroy sums it up: "Pornography benefits women, both personally and politically. . . . Historically, feminism and pornography have been fellow travelers on the rocky road of unorthodoxy. This partnership was natural, perhaps inevitable. After all, both feminism and pornography flout the traditional notion that sex is necessarily connected to marriage or procreation. Both view women as sexual beings who should pursue their sexuality for pleasure and self-fulfillment. Indeed, most of feminism's demands have been phrased in terms of women's sexuality: equal marriage, lesbianism, birth control, abortion, gender justice."[3] And for McElroy, the similarities don't end there. Both feminism and pornography flourish when there is an atmosphere of tolerance, and when there is respect for dissident positions and attitudes. Likewise, both feminism and pornography are repressed when sexual expression is censored and regulated. Because freedom of expression is freedom to demand change, the benefits of free expression are greater for those who want to reform society than for those who want to maintain the status quo.

PORN

Is it possible to make feminist porn? I definitely think so. Pornography contains a discourse, just like any other kind of cultural or artistic expression. In pornography's case, the discourse involves sex, and whatever contains a discourse can be approached from a feminist point of view.

If women don't take a role as creators of pornography's discourse, then porn won't express anything but what men think about sex. We should take part to explain what we're like, what our sexuality is like, and what our experience of sex is like. If we leave it all to men, porn will keep representing us the way we're seen in male fantasy—as whores, Lolitas, nymphomaniacs, and all the other stereotypes we've already mentioned.

Besides, the cliché about the adult film industry—that the settings and the treatment of women are usually degrading—is based on common practices that are fairly widespread among male producers and directors. My friend Audacia Ray, a director of adult films, has this to say: "To me, making feminist porn is not about what is actually shown on screen and much more about what is happening on the production end of things. . . . Does that performer want to be there? Is the director/producer respecting her needs and paying her appropriately? Did she get blindsided by requests for acts she doesn't want to do? The answers to those questions determine whether or not the porn is feminist, sex-positive, and ethical for me, not what is happening on screen."[4]

X-Rated Feminist Films = X-Rated Antisexist Films
Feminist Pizza Boy

What does it take for an adult film to be feminist? I like to answer that question by saying it's enough if the film simply isn't sexist. Consider my first short, *The Good Girl*, which I shot in 2004. I decided to film that old chestnut about the pizza delivery guy, but from a woman's viewpoint. Basically, men have constructed this fantasy as follows: the delivery guy arrives with the pizza, the girl smiles at him, he asks her for the money, she doesn't have it, he gets mad, she smiles again and takes off her clothes, he relaxes, enjoys a good blow job, fucks her, comes, and goes away happy. Any sexism here? I certainly think so—the girl is foolish, she's a whore, she's easy, and the guy is happy trading sex for money.

But *The Good Girl* was conceived from a woman's point of view. It's a story about the feelings of a young woman who is playing with her sexual fantasies. She is the one at the center of this short film, she is the one moving the action forward, and she is the one choosing to live out her porn fantasy. It's archetypal porn, all the way to the grand finale, in which the delivery guy comes on her face, but that's something she herself wants, and it happens only after she's had her orgasm. The very title of this short is a metaphor for what it means to be a "good" girl. And the woman isn't "whorified," either—she pays for her pizza, and she even offers the guy a postcoital slice.

For me, though, a kinky lesbian scene between a pregnant Belladonna and her girlfriend also counts as feminist porn, since no sexist ideology is being reproduced on the screen, she's acting freely, and there's no male power holding her down.

I Don't Have All the Answers

A lot of men (and some women) ask me, "Who are you to say what women like? Who are you to say what's feminist or not?" And I agree with them

100 percent—neither I nor anyone else should be claiming to lay down the rules for adult films. Every woman is different, and I certainly don't think I have the answers for all women. That's why I think we need all kinds of women giving expression to their own individual visions. But if anything at all is for sure, it's that all of us women share the experience of being women. As Lucía Etxebarría has written, "The society in which we live has a defining influence on the construction of desire, fantasies, and sexual imagery. And because men and women, unfortunately, are brought up and socialized in different ways, our ways of experiencing sex, and thus of writing about it, will necessarily also be different."[5]

> *The new adult boutiques, "Tuppersex" parties, deluxe new sex toys, porn for women—all of it expresses the liberation of today's woman, a sexual consumer as free and active as men have been for centuries.*

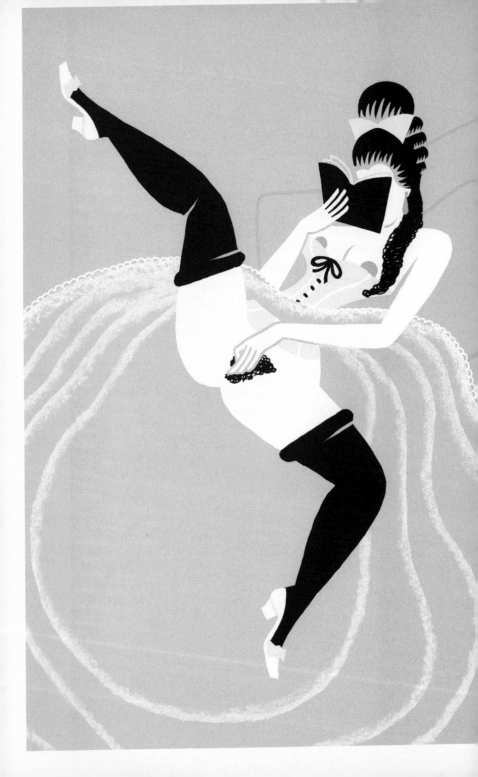

CHAPTER 3
THE HISTORY OF PORN

The difference between the Venuses of the Stone Age and the age of PornoTube is not just a matter of some twenty-four thousand years. There have also been big changes in the meanings and intentions of erotic imagery. But its essence has continued unchanged—sex, sex, and more sex. Becoming familiar with the history of eroticism and pornography across the ages can help us get oriented and improve our understanding of how we ended up where we are.

The word *pornographic* actually comes from two Greek words, *pornē* ("prostitute") and *graphein* ("to write"), whose literal meaning adds up to "writing about a prostitute." In this chapter, we'll use the term "erotic" in referring to pre-Victorian works of a sexual nature, since it was only in the Victorian era that the term "pornography" was coined.

PALEOLITHIC PORN
The first erotic images to come down to us from history were created in the Paleolithic era. They are basically figurines of naked human beings with exaggerated sexual features, a symbol of fertility in the female figurines. Two clear examples of such figurines are the Willendorf and Malta Venuses, also known as the "immodest" Venuses.[1] They were made not for erotic stimulation but for use in

religious rituals, since fertility was a concept that also applied to the earth and its generosity with fruits of the harvest and the hunt. And so we know that in pre-Christian times, before sex came to be associated with sin and prohibition, erotic images had a distinct spiritual meaning.

GREECE: SMALL IS BEAUTIFUL

At the high point of their culture, the Greeks were working with a concept of erotica much closer to our own, as can be seen in their works. Ancient Greek ceramic plates and sculptures contain the first homosexual imagery in recorded history (that's why the term *Greek* is used in connection with anal sex), and there are also plates that feature images of adults having sex with very young boys. Today we would see such images as examples of pederasty and hardcore porn, but let's not forget that we're talking about a time several centuries before the invention of sin. Phallic imagery was quite common, since phallic symbols were thought to be protective. A clear example of such imagery is seen in the Herma of Demosthenes, a figure dating from 280 B.C.E, which probably stood in a marketplace. It consists of a bust of Hermes carved into the top of a block of stone, and carved into the lower portion of the stone is a set of male genitals that people anointed with olive oil to attract good luck. The Greek ideal of beauty was a man with a small penis, an ideal later adopted by the Romans. Nacho Vidal certainly is lucky to have been born when he was!

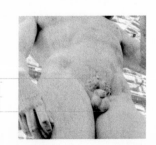

RECOMMENDED DOCUMENTARY

PORNOGRAPHY: THE SECRET HISTORY OF CIVILIZATION

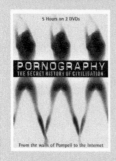

You might expect a documentary on the history of pornography to be fairly playful and erotic, and to use the documentary concept as little more than a playful excuse for showing naked people. But that's not the case here. I highly recommend this profound, intelligent series by Fenton Bailey and Randy Barbato, who also directed *Inside Deep Throat*, the other documentary recommended in this chapter. In this work, which covers a thousand years of pornographic history in five hours, we learn from art and film historians, experts on sexuality, and even a few sex workers like Marilyn Chambers and John Leslie that porn is anything but a recent, twentieth-century invention.

Writer and director: Fenton Bailey and Randy Barbato
Country: United States
Year: 2000
Time: 5 hours
Genre: Documentary series (6 episodes)

ROME: *HIC HABITAT FELICITAS*

In the painting and sculpture of the ancient Roman Empire there are also plenty of erotic references, some of them in Pompeii's world-famous Villa dei Misteri, or Villa of Mysteries, which is decorated with frescoes that, thanks to the eruption of Mount Vesuvius, have been relatively well preserved. One such fresco, in the Villa's *triclinium*, shows a woman being whipped. Most theorists believe that the practice of whipping belonged to the initiatory

45

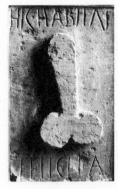

rites of a secret cult devoted to the god Dionysus, although the French archaeologist Paul Veyne maintains that whipping formed part of a marriage ritual.

Phallic imagery continued to be the order of the day, in terms of both decoration (phalluses were felt to represent the height of good taste) and direction (that is, a phallus indicated the presence of a whorehouse). Prostitution has been called the world's oldest profession, and that seems about right. But the Roman whorehouses held none of the implicitly negative connotations that whorehouses have today. A whorehouse was simply a place of leisure, as healthy and valid as a modern football stadium or amusement park.

On one of the most famous stone tablets showing a *fascinus* (a Roman word meaning "phallus,"[2] presumably the root of our word "fascinate," given its supposedly magical connotations), the relief figure of a penis is accompanied by the words *Hic habitat felicitas* ("Here lives happiness"), a figure presumably placed on the door of a house to attract good luck. And on the wall of a Pompeii whorehouse is what could be regarded as the world's first piece of graffiti—a tablet reading *Hic bene futuit* ("Here I had a great fuck"). Not a bad marketing strategy!

ORGIES OF THE ORIENT

Far Eastern cultures, too, have an abundant tradition of erotic art. Japan and China, like India and Persia, harbor a great many works joyfully celebrating humanity's art of love. For example, the *Kama Sutra*, the first sex manual in recorded history, came from India, where it was written by

Mallanaga Vatsyayana, most likely around the second century C.E. The book is commonly regarded as the first written work of pornography, but in reality it's more like a do-it-yourself manual. It mixes advice about the sixty-four "arts" (activities, such as dancing, writing, drawing, magic, and sorcery, that might possibly accompany the sex act) with instructions intended to help the reader become a model citizen—or seduce the wives of fellow citizens. The book, as comprehensive as they come, is adorned with detailed, hand-drawn explanatory illustrations of every single position, some of them more appropriate for a contortionist than a pleasure seeker.

Eleventh-century India saw the completion of one of the world's most famous repositories of erotic sculpture—the Khajuraho Temples, made of granite and built between approximately 950 and 1050 C.E. The sculptures housed in the temples depict not only animals, flowers, and plants but also people making love in various positions. The intention behind the latter group of sculptures isn't clear today. Some believe their intention was educational, and that the sculptures were meant to teach the sexual positions of the *Kama Sutra*, whereas others say that the sculptures portray an orgy of sorts, in honor of the divine union between Shiva and Parvati.

The Japanese have a special designation for a certain kind of erotic painting—*shunga*, which can be translated as "picture of spring," the word

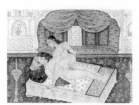 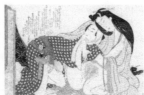 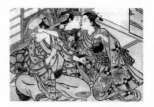

spring being a typical euphemism for coitus. These paintings, inspired by the illustrative plates in medical books, began to appear in the seventh century C.E., and they depict scenes of heterosexual and homosexual encounters incorporating every conceivable position. With their realist aesthetic, *shunga* portray ordinary life. They were never regarded as minor works, nor were they seen as dirty. On the contrary, even the most important artists painted *shunga* at the height of this genre's production. Sometimes the figures have exaggerated genitals, but only for the sake of visibility, given the small proportions of these works. *Shunga*, which also take the form of handmade statuettes (*netsuke* carvings), continued to be produced into the nineteenth century, until they were eclipsed by the popularity of pornographic photography.

THE MIDDLE AGES: SEX AMONG THE PSALMS

The European Middle Ages are also known as the Dark Ages because of the way the whole era, especially the early years, was laid waste by the negative influence that religion exercised over art. But even the Middle Ages were not without erotic representations. These took the form of miniatures, small drawings or paintings that, oddly enough, were added to the margins of handmade psalm books and religious texts. Thus erotic art ceased for the first time to be the popular genre it had been for the Greeks and Romans and became instead a luxury available only to the privileged, moneyed few.

The year 1398 stands out as a very important date in the history of pornography. This is thought to be the birth date of Johannes Gutenberg, the German printer recognized as the first European to print from movable type. As such, Gutenberg is credited not only with democratizing literature but also with spreading pornography all over the West, a project aided, some five centuries later, by the appearance of the daguerrotype. In fact, any technological advance that has ever facilitated the transmission of information has also been a step forward in the spread of pornography. The Internet has now made pornography more popular than ever, but Gutenberg took the first, giant step.

RACY RENAISSANCE NOVELS

Naked bodies were a fixture in Renaissance art, but their function wasn't entirely erotic. They were also understood to be faithful representations of nature, in keeping with a characteristic motif of that period. But the Roman Catholic Church still held enough power for Pope Clement VII to have the first publisher of *I Modi* thrown in jail. This album of erotic drawings, also known as *The Sixteen Pleasures*, is unfortunately renowned for the harassment directed its way during the sixteenth century. After the original edition of *I Modi* was burned, anyone who dared to publish a new edition was threatened with imprisonment, and so a market developed for a series of copies that identified neither the publisher nor the illustrator. These copies became the first underground porn in recorded history.

Starting in the seventeenth century, novels that can be considered the precursors of pornographic literature began to appear regularly in Europe. (Although the "Song of Solomon" includes lines that could make a porn starlet blush, this book of the Old Testament is not considered an erotic novel.) Foremost among these novels are the French *L'École des filles ou La philosophie des dames* and the Italian *La Puttana errante*. They cover much the same ground as a modern novel, since very little about sex has changed over the past few centuries.

The English novel *Fanny Hill* deserves special mention. Written in 1784 as social criticism, it nevertheless makes playful use of erotic scenes featuring its female narrator. Because the novel piles euphemism on euphemism, the sex acts exist only in the reader's mind, but that was still enough to land its author in jail. More than two hundred years later, *Fanny Hill* remains one of the most translated and best-selling English novels of all time.

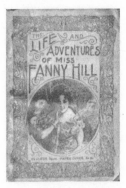

Victorian literature, too, includes a large number of pornographic works, despite the era's prevailing repression. One of the most interesting is *My Secret Life* (1890), which portrays the underbelly of a puritanical society while taking full advantage of the opportunity to relate the sexual adventures of a young Englishman in lavish detail.

PHOTOGRAPHY AND FILM: NEW INVENTIONS AT PORN'S FINGERTIPS

They say that when photography was invented, in 1827, and when movies were invented, in 1894, five minutes later a naked woman must have been striking a pose for the camera.

The first cinematic instance of a woman disrobing came in 1896, when the French film *Le Bain* showed the

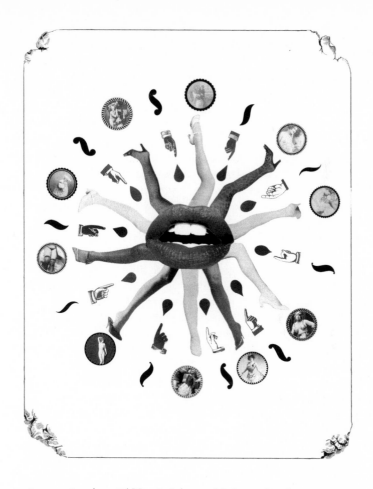

actress Louise Willy taking off her clothes to step into a bathtub—an exercise in naiveté, as far as we're concerned, but it did mark a "before" and an "after" in the history of erotica. Before long, the German producer Oskar Messter had released a series of films showing unclad women performing gymnastics, bathing, and dancing. These films were the precursors of stag movies—films made exclusively for men and shown in bordellos or at private screenings and bachelor parties.

Exploitation films were born in the early 1920s when Louis Sonney, an Italian immigrant and the sheriff of small-town Centralia, Washington, took his reward money for capturing the "smiling bandit," a train robber named Roy Gardner, and made a movie warning about the dangers of a life of crime. Once he discovered the potential of this format, he decided to focus on the dangers of sex (illustrating his points, of course, with appropriate scenes), and it was these dangers that prompted him to make more than four hundred films, which were very well received by fans of the genre.

The same era saw the publication of *Lady Chatterley's Lover*, written by D. H. Lawrence between 1926 and 1927 and classified as pornography, which meant that the novel in unexpurgated form was banned in England as well as in the United States. In 1959, a federal judge overturned the ban in the United States, citing the quality of the work (today considered a masterpiece of world literature) and the author's genius.

Soon porn was revolutionized by yet another invention—the 8mm projector, which opened the door to amateur porn and movies made to order for rich men and aristocrats. Because most of these films starred prostitutes and were shot in bordellos, their production costs were quite low, and they were fairly affordable. Now it was possible to watch pornography in the privacy of one's home, and this gave new meaning to the genre.

The 1950s brought the popularization of nudie flicks, featuring striptease and burlesque scenes that had little to do with porn. Softcore elements like simulated sex began to be added, and Russ Meyer released *The Immoral Mr. Teas*, his first commercially successful film.

In the 1960s, with the famously strict Hays Code in force in the United States, the world capital of pornographic film was Copenhagen. The Hays Code imposed tight restrictions on nudity, bedroom scenes, references to homosexuality, and even kisses thought to be excessively passionate. The porn capital moved to the United States in 1966, when the Hays Code was abolished. As a curious historical note, the opening shots in the battle against the Hays Code were fired not on behalf of film production companies but by Hugh Hefner on behalf of *Playboy*, whose pages juxtaposed articles of great social and cultural interest with images of seminude women.

The post-Hays era brought a new classification for movies—the X rating, reserved for films that serve up big helpings of sex and violence. The first X-rated film to be screened in mainstream[3] movie theaters was *Mona: The Virgin Nymph* (1970), though its success was soon eclipsed by that of *Deep Throat*, released just two years later.

THE GOLDEN AGE OF PORN

The golden age of pornographic films had begun, bringing with it an astounding array of high-quality titles like *The Devil in Miss Jones*, *Behind the Green Door*, *Debbie Does Dallas*, *Emmanuelle*, and other top X-rated releases in which sex shared the screen with humor and good dialogue, a combination that later on would become difficult to find again in this genre.

The 1980s brought the home VCR and widespread access to adult films, which until then could be viewed only in adult theaters. The demand grew, and so did the supply. The films became more and more rushed, and less and less creative, and as the genre moved into mass production, filmmakers stopped making pornographic movies and simply made pornographic videos, with the loss of quality that

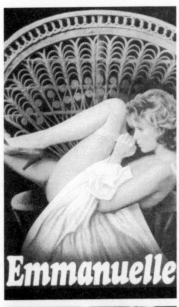

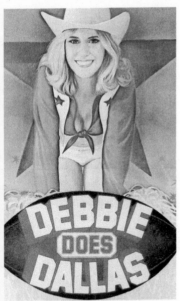

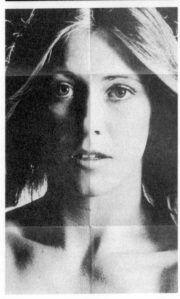

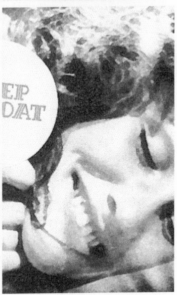

such a change entails. Fortunately, the burgeoning popularity of adult film festivals did manage to enliven an industry that went through whole periods in which not a single memorable film was produced. The best thing that happened to porn in the 1980s was Femme Productions, founded by Candida Royalle, a former porn actress, and with Femme came X-rated films for couples, which can be regarded as the first step toward a feminist porn.

In the 1990s, performers in porn films began to be seen again as stars, a status they hadn't enjoyed since the 1970s. This decade also marked the beginning of the era of big-budget porn films and the transformation of porn workers into popular icons. Who hasn't heard of Traci Lords, Ron Jeremy, Jenna Jameson, Asia Carrera, and Rocco Siffredi? You don't have to be a big porn fan to recognize their names and faces.

THE INTERNET

With the growing popularity of the Internet and the widespread availability of broadband—crucial to porn, since it allows high-speed viewing and downloading of images (real torture over a 52k modem)—the first decade of the twenty-first century has brought us do-it-yourself porn. Now anyone, in a matter of minutes, can become the star of his or her own filmed erotic fantasies and share them online.

But the truly remarkable thing about the adult film scene over the past few years is the fact that women are starting to take center stage, not only as porn consumers, but also as porn professionals, going beyond acting in porn and beginning to produce and direct films that are a breath of fresh air for the genre.

RECOMMENDED DOCUMENTARY

INSIDE DEEP THROAT

It was a low-budget, $25,000 production that became a $600 million phenomenon.[4] It provoked an administration to declare war on the First Amendment.[5] It made buying a movie ticket a revolutionary act. Generally considered the highest-grossing movie of all time, the 1972 adult film *Deep Throat* was more than a stimulating curiosity, more than a box-office triumph. Released at the moment when nationwide movements for sexual freedom, equal rights, and countercultural values were reaching their peak, this sexually explicit film abruptly became the epicenter of an unprecedented sociopolitical earthquake, a huge cultural phenomenon whose impact is still felt today. Now, nearly four decades after *Deep Throat* burst into the collective imagination, this documentary examines the gulf between the filmmakers' modest intentions and the surprising legacy they never intended to leave.

Writer and director: Fenton Bailey and Randy Barbato
Country: United States
Year: 2005
Time: 92 minutes
Genre: Documentary

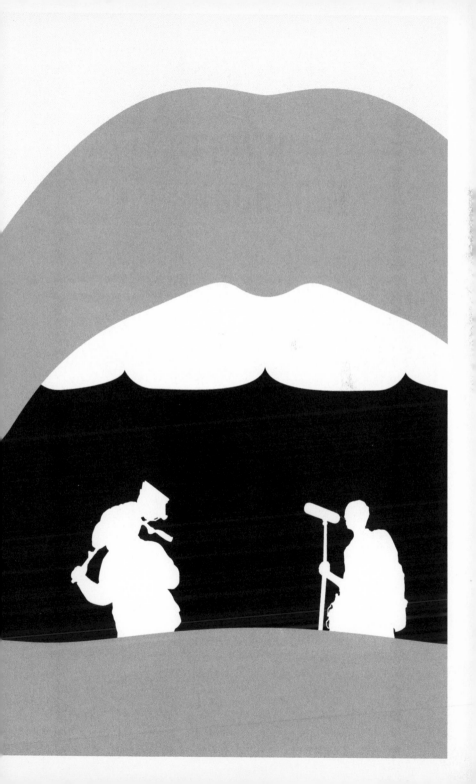

CHAPTER 4

FAQs

I've already mentioned that women tend to be much less informed about porn than men are, so in this chapter I've pulled together the questions that come up most often on chat boards, in interviews, and in my email, and I've answered them to give you a better idea of what the porn industry is all about.

1. Do pornographic films exploit women?

Sasha Grey, one of the hippest of a new breed of U.S. porn actresses, answers this question by saying that even though plenty of people think of her as a victim, she has never been sexually abused by anyone. She also denies taking drugs, and she claims never to have done anything for the camera that she didn't want to do. She believes very strongly in what she's doing, and she wants women to know that it's all right to have twisted fantasies and adventurous sex. Women, she says, don't have to be ladies in bed.

2. How can I be sure that nobody in an X-rated film is a minor or was forced to participate?

Every year, a ton of money is made in the adult film industry—a legal, highly regulated business. These days a pornographic film production can't go forward unless it's possible to verify the identities of all the performers and prove that they're all of legal age. Every performer has to sign a model release, too. These measures guarantee that there has been no coercion of any kind, and that the actors and actresses are working because they enjoy it and it suits them financially.

3. How much money is there in porn, and how many adult films are made every year?

About fourteen thousand adult films are released every year. And that's just the ones we know about, because today there's also a lot of other material being produced, not as movies for the adult film market but as single scenes for the Internet. According to *Adult Video News (AVN)*, the trade magazine of the adult film industry, pornographic films pull in some $3 billion per year, but this is one sector that's hard to measure, since actual earnings may be quite a bit higher. As in the mainstream film industry, the largest producer of pornographic films by far is the United States.

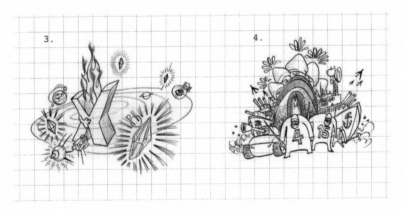

4. What kinds of preventive measures are taken to avoid STDs?

All kinds of prevention are used, the same as in real life. Blood tests for STDs are required of all performers, and these tests must be documented in a film's production records. Testing is conducted regularly, to keep the performers informed about their health. Condoms should be used as well, but sometimes market demand prevails instead.

5. Why is there sex between women but never between men?

Traditional porn is made for straight men, and sex between men is somehow seen as an attack against manhood. But all the "out" women in adult movies are potentially bisexual—that's what turns guys on. It also means that women can be fucked two at a time.

6. Why do the men always ejaculate outside?

Ejaculation is the be-all and end-all of masculinity, life, and everything else. That's why it's traditionally shown in male-oriented porn, as proof of orgasm and the man's sexual enjoyment.

7. Why are there so few women directing adult films?

The porn industry was created principally by men and for men, so it's not a business that women can easily break into except in minor roles. Clearly, though, things are improving, now that a few independent producers—women making films for women—are fighting to change things.

8. What's the difference between eroticism and pornography?

In theory, the difference is that genitals are not concealed in pornography, whereas everything in

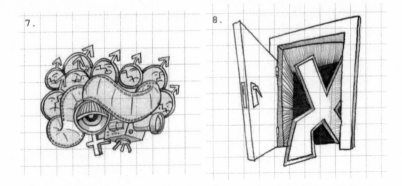

eroticism is subtle, and the sex is only implied. I don't really think it's that cut and dried, however. I think the line between eroticism and pornography, like the way each is defined, has to do primarily with the ethics and tastes of whoever is watching the images in question. What the two have in common, though, is the goal of turning us on, and one genre does that more graphically and more explicitly than the other.

9. What has AIDS meant for the porn industry?

In the first wave of the pandemic, AIDS claimed a number of performers, some of them big stars like John Holmes. Today there are comprehensive checks in place, with blood tests required on a regular basis. Anyone who tests positive for HIV is immediately banned from working as a performer.

10. Who are your favorite porn actors and actresses, and where do you find them?

I like natural-looking guys and girls, not your typical Nacho or Rocco or Jenna Jameson. Barcelona, where I live, is a gold mine of young performers, but I also use agencies in Prague, Budapest, and London, cities that also have very good actors and actresses.

11. After the director yells "Cut," does the action ever continue?

No. Shooting an adult film is much more technical than it is entertaining. The guys and girls are very professional, and they're on the set to make a movie. Obviously, if the atmosphere is right, the sex will be enjoyable, but as a rule the performers are strictly professional, and they don't want to hang around the set making out after the director yells "Cut!" They'd rather get up and take a shower.

12. Does anybody perform in adult films just to get off?

In theory, acting in a professional pornographic film is work. In homemade and amateur porn, of course, there are lots of people doing it just to get off.

13. Do fluffers really exist?

They used to. A fluffer was someone, almost always a woman, whose job it was to keep the male performers turned on between scenes. These days, guys are required to be ready to go without needing anyone else to touch them. They have to be self-starters and get it up without assistance of any kind.

14. And how does a male actor manage to keep it up?

On the theory that an adult film actor is a professional sex worker, it's assumed that he can exercise control over his body in general and his penis in particular. But if theory lets him down, he can always turn for help to Viagra, the little blue miracle pill that will get him hard in minutes.

15. I'd like to act in a porn film, but I don't want my face to be seen. Is that possible?

No, it isn't. All pornographic movies show the face, since the face is a part of the body that can be used to show the sexual pleasure that the performers are assumed to be feeling. Anyway, it's necessary to show the face in scenes featuring oral sex, which occurs in 99.9 percent of adult films.

16. Do porn actresses fake orgasms?

Yes, most of the time. It's possible, though, for an actress to have a real orgasm, depending on the girl, the shoot, and the other actors or actresses who happen to be touching her in a particular scene. And why shouldn't it be possible for a porn actress to come for real? In this industry above all, business really ought to mix with pleasure.

17. Are there secrets to producing more sperm and standing out in the money shots?

Yes. These secrets can be found on the Internet, under the names Virilix and Volume 500. Products like these are usually a blend of natural plant extracts that enhance the quantity and quality of sperm in addition to promoting sexual vitality overall.

18. How much money do performers usually make for a shoot or a scene?

In Europe, an actress usually gets between five hundred and fifteen hundred euros per scene, depending on such factors as her fame, her cachet, and the scene's complexity. Guys earn somewhat less, between three hundred and one thousand euros per scene.

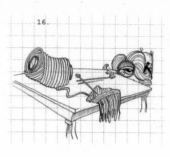

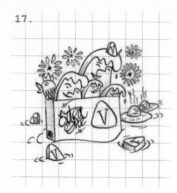

19. Is it true that only actors with eight inches need apply?

Even though size does matter in this business, it isn't really a deal breaker. A big beautiful cock doesn't hurt, of course, but you'll get by with one that can get hard and stay hard when it needs to.

20. I want to act in adult films? What should I do?

First of all, I suggest that you film a scene with your partner, and get yourself some good photos showing your face and your whole body. Then, if you're still comfortable and want to take the next step, you can approach one of the talent agencies that normally do this kind of casting. Such agencies exist in most of the world's major cities.

21. Do porn actresses work as prostitutes?

Usually it's the other way around—some call girls make pornographic movies as a way to attract more clients or enhance their own cachet—but it's important to understand that being a porn actress is not the same as being a prostitute.

22. Will watching porn online leave traces on my computer?

Pages on porn sites are usually loaded with cookies—fragments of code that get stored on your

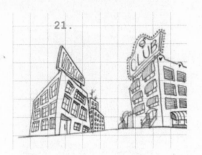

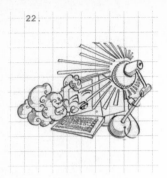

hard drive via your browser—and even Trojan Horse viruses install themselves on your system to track you online. But they shouldn't be a problem if you have a good antivirus program. Besides, you can always click your browser's "history" tab and erase your tracks from time to time.

23. Can watching porn make you a pervert?

According to *Merriam-Webster's 11th Collegiate Dictionary*, *to pervert* means "to cause to turn aside or away from what is good or true or morally right." Porn won't do that to you, but it may be able to spice up your sexual imagination and make you naughtier.

24. Are there any long-term couples in the world of adult film?

Yes, there are. As professionals, though, they have to be able to set jealousy and possessiveness aside when a partner is shooting scenes with other people. Those scenes are just perks of the job. They have nothing to do with infidelity.

25. Is it healthy to watch porn and masturbate even though you have a partner?

Whether you have a partner or not, masturbation is always healthy because it gives you pleasure and helps you know what you like. If you watch porn while you're masturbating, you can get ideas to try out later with your partner and surprise him or her with some interesting new tricks. Sexual fantasies are our greatest treasure! If we nurture them, they'll make us even better lovers.

26. Are there any adult films made just for women?

Yes, there are. Basically, films like these have a positive image of women. They don't degrade women or treat women like whores or victims. They accept women as active sexual beings. These films are visually interesting, and their dialogue and plots are interesting as well. And of course men can watch these films, too—everyone is invited to this party!

27. What was the greatest moment in the history of pornographic film?

The 1970s, also known as the golden age of porn. That was when the best movies were made, when adult films crossed over into mainstream theaters, and when porn stars were treated like real celebrities.

28. My partner wants us to watch an adult film together, but I'm embarrassed. What should I do?

To begin with, watching an adult film with your partner should be fun, not a reason to feel embarrassed or ashamed or not have a good time. So start off by looking for a film just for you, and when you find one you like, a film you feel comfortable with, look for a scene that really turns you on, and then suggest to your partner that the two of you have dinner—with a surprise for dessert!

29. My boyfriend wants us to do a homemade porn movie together. How can I be sure I won't end up all over the Internet?

There's only one way to be sure—don't let the video or digital master out of your hands, and don't let him make any copies. This means you'll be the one making the movie, and you'll be the one keeping the master. You can watch the movie with him whenever you like, but the master will always be under your control.

30. Where can I buy or watch good pornographic films?

This book contains lots of information about that, but if you want to locate the sources closest to where you live, Google "sex toys" or "adult boutiques" along with the name of your city, and you're bound to find some interesting choices. Otherwise, there's always an online store, which can quickly and very discreetly get adult films to you at home.

31.
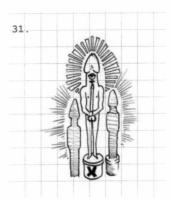

32.
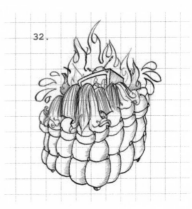

31. Does porn have anything like the Oscars?

There are more and more local and regional porn festivals, but the closest thing porn has to the Oscars is the AVN Awards, which take place in Las Vegas in conjunction with the Adult Entertainment Expo, the adult film world's biggest event. Prizes are awarded in more than a hundred different categories, and a win can double someone's cachet or cause sales to skyrocket—the dream of every actor and director in adult films.

32. Do women normally watch porn?

We certainly do, even though many of us don't realize that we're watching porn, or we have trouble admitting it. In the 1990s, in fact, with the advent of cable and satellite TV, the biggest consumers of porn were discovered to be housewives making the best of their free time while their husbands were at the office and their children were at school.

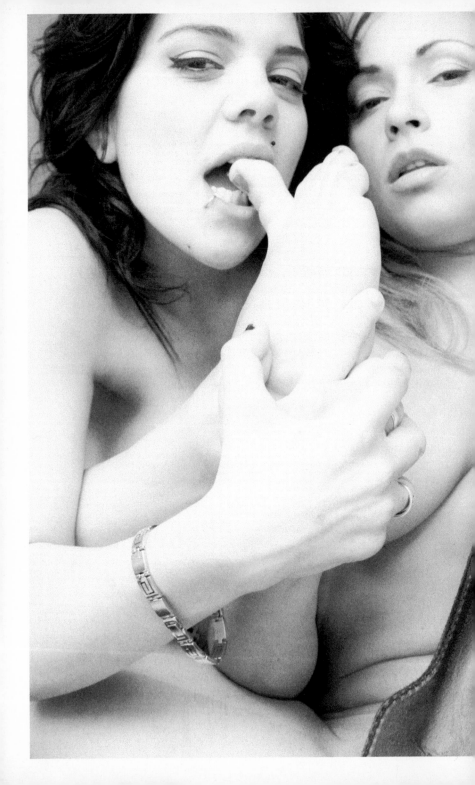

CHAPTER 5
A DICTIONARY OF PORN

----

alt-porn *n.* independently created pornography

anal *adj. 1.* pertaining to the anus 2. (short form of *anal sex*) penetration of the anus in general, whether with the penis, the fingers, or sex toys

analingus: *see* rim job

BDSM *n.* (acronym for *bondage, discipline, and sado-masochism*) dominant-submissive sex play in general

bisexual: *adj.* 1. possessing attributes of both sexes; hermaphroditic 2. of, relating to, or characterized by a tendency to direct sexual desire toward both sexes *n.* in traditional porn, a term synonymous with *woman*

blow job *n.* oral sex performed on a man

bondage *n.* in dominant-submissive sex play, the use of certain kinds of clothing or devices to restrict movement

bubblegum *n.* a term used in the adult film industry to denote an especially pink vagina

bukkake *n.* (reputedly from Japanese *bukkakeru*, said to denote the act of dashing or sloshing water on a person or in a person's face) the practice—described by some sources as being of ancient origin, whereas others dismiss that claim as an urban legend—in which men in a group (supposedly numbering from ten to one hundred) ejaculate together on one woman

CFNM *n.* (acronym for *clothed female, nude male*) a practice in which a woman who is more or less clothed abuses a completely naked man

cock ring *n.* a ring of metal, leather, or rubber worn around the testicles and penis to prolong erection and delay ejaculation

cowgirl *adj.* a term describing a face-to-face sexual position (*woman on top*) in which the man lies on his back and the woman mounts him (a woman facing the man's feet assumes the *reverse cowgirl* position)

cream pie *n.* ejaculated semen that a woman expels from her vagina with the use of her pelvic-floor muscles

cum *n.* semen

cunnilingus *n.* oral sex performed on a woman

dildo *n.* a penis-shaped object generally used for vaginal or anal masturbation

doggy style *n.* a sexual position in which a woman is on her hands and knees and a partner penetrates her from behind

double penetration *n.* a sexual scenario in which the participants are two men (or two sex toys) and one woman, and whose three possible variations are both penises (toys) in the woman's vagina, both penises (toys) in the woman's anus, or one penis (toy) in the woman's vagina and one in her anus

English discipline *n.* dominant-submissive sex play, primarily mild and verbal but possibly including the use of whipping or caning

exhibitionism *n.* 1. the urge to expose one's genitals to others, especially strangers 2. the act of taking pleasure in exhibiting one's body in lewd positions or having sex in public

facial *n.* the practice, very common in pornographic films since the 1990s, of a male actor ejaculating on his partner's face

feminist porn *n.* a genre of pornography primarily created by and for women

fetishism *n.* the practice of fixating on a particular body part, or on an item associated with it, as the object of sexual excitement and desire

fisting *n.* partial or complete insertion of the fist into a partner's anus or vagina

gang bang *n.* a group scenario, including a theoretically indefinite number of participants, in which a woman has sex with one person after another

girl-on-girl *adj.* in a pornographic film, pertaining to a scene that features sexual contact between two women

gonzo *adj.* (from the name of a type of journalism, pioneered by Hunter S. Thompson, in which the writer becomes a participant in the events on which he or she is reporting) a term describing pornography in which the camera operator or the director participates in the action

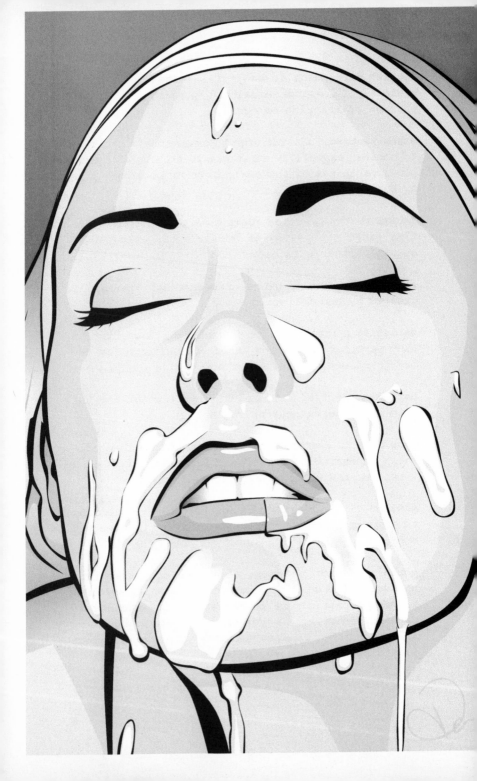

hardcore *adj.* containing explicit representations of sex acts or actual sex acts

hermaphrodite *n.* (from *Hermaphroditus*, proper name of the son of Hermes and Aphrodite, who in the legend recounted by Ovid was so loved by the nymph Salmacis that she prayed for complete union with him, with the result that they were united in one body combining male and female characteristics) someone who possesses attributes of both sexes

interracial *adj.* in a pornographic film, a term describing a scene that features people of different races, but usually referring to a scene using both white and African American participants

IP (acronym for *internal popshot*) in pornography, the fairly unusual practice of ejaculation inside the vagina

kokigami *n.* (from the Japanese word *koki*, a small piece of cloth worn at the waist by *waki*, the supporting actors in *Noh* drama, and the Japanese word *gami*, paper) the Japanese art of dressing the erect penis in little paper costumes or disguises, such as that of a dragon or some other animal

latex *n.* a plastic-type material dear to many fetishists and often used in pornographic productions

mainstream porn *n.* the type of male-oriented porn that most people watch nowadays on VCRs and online, and which began to be produced in the 1980s, with the appearance of home video and VCRs (the term *mainstream*, originally a noun denoting the principal current of a river and now defined by *Webster's 11th Collegiate Dictionary* as "a prevailing current or direction of activity or influence," was first used as an adjective in connection with art and music and gradually came to describe popular culture of all kinds)

masturbation *n.* stimulation of the genitals or erogenous zones by hand or by other means to give sexual pleasure

medical shot *n.* in a pornographic film, a close-up of genitals in action, shown either by themselves or together with one or more additional sets of genitals

MET Art *n.* (from *MET*, acronym for *most erotic teens*, and *art*) 1. a website (www.met-art.com) featuring erotic photographs or videos with artistic pretensions, in which the subjects, who appear to be adolescents, may or may not actually be adolescents but in any case are always of legal age 2. erotic photographs or videos of this kind

MILF *n.* (acronym for *mother I'd like to fuck*) a genre of pornography featuring sex with attractive mature women

missionary *adj.* pertaining or relating to a standard face-to-face sexual position in which the man lies on top of the woman, who is on her back with her legs spread

mistress *n.* dominatrix; a woman who takes the dominant role in a dominant-submissive or sadomasochistic relationship

money shot *n.* in a pornographic film, the shot in which a male actor ejaculates (and thus earns his fee)

mummification *n.* a bondage technique that consists

76

of restraining a person by completely wrapping his or her body in materials ranging from Saran Wrap to bandages

orgy *n.* in a pornographic film, a scene that includes five or more people as well as multiple changes of partners (pairs, threesomes, and so on)

paraphilia *n.* a pattern of sexual behavior in which satisfaction is found not in intercourse but in some other activity, or in things that may range from reptiles to music

pinup *n.* an aesthetic of female glamour based on 1950s pinups, especially those featuring the actress and stripper Bettie Page

porn star *n.* an actor or an actress who has achieved movie-star status in pornographic films

POV *adj.* (acronym for *point of view*) pertaining or relating to a type of homemade pornographic movie filmed from the point of view of a man holding a camera

rim job *n.* the practice of licking the anus and/or penetrating the anus with the tongue; rimming

sadomasochism (S&M) *n.* (from the surnames of the Marquis de *Sade*, a French novelist, and the Austrian novelist Leopold von Sacher-*Masoch*, both of whose works depict sexual relationships based on a dialectic of master and slave) the act of taking pleasure in inflicting physical or mental pain either on others or on oneself

shibari *n.* a style of Japanese bondage carried out as a very refined sexual practice

slave *n.* a man or a woman who plays the submissive role in a sadomasochistic relationship

snowballing *n.* 1. the practice of kissing a woman after ejaculating on her face 2. the practice of passing semen that has been ejaculated into one's mouth into the mouth of another person

softcore *n.* a mild form of pornography containing neither explicit representations of sex nor penetration

squirting *n.* female ejaculation

striptease *n.* a form of sensual dance in which a performer undresses to musical accompaniment, more or less gracefully and with more or less charm

threesome *n.* a sexual encounter involving three participants in varying opposite- and same-sex configurations

Viagra *n.* a compound (sildenafil citrate) synthesized by Pfizer in 1996 that promotes erection of the penis through vasoconstriction and is used in the treatment of erectile dysfunction

vibrator *n.* a type of sex toy, often a dildo, that uses a vibrating mechanism to intensify sexual sensations

webcam n. a digital audiovisual device connected to a computer and widely used in recording pornographic home videos as well as in practicing Internet-based exhibitionism

yoga porn *n.* a genre of porn featuring a man's oral stimulation of his own penis

yogi *n.* in pornography, a man capable of performing fellatio on himself

zoophilia *n.* practices that include having sex with animals; bestiality

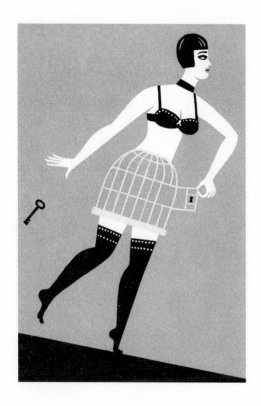

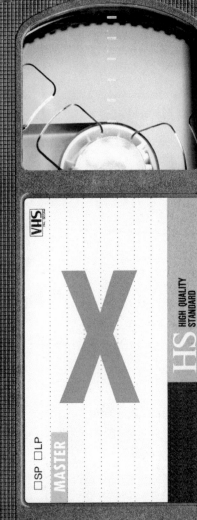
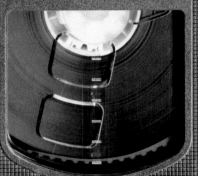

CHAPTER 6
HORROR MOVIES, COMEDIES, AND PORN

I like to think of porn as just one more type of audiovisual entertainment, and I often compare it to other types of films, such as horror movies and comedies. Just as horror movies want to scare you to death, and comedies want to get you rolling in the aisle, porn wants to turn you on.

Every viewer is different. A friend of yours might recommend a comedy that had her on the floor, but you see it and feel like crying. Or maybe you hear about some horror film that's supposed to scare the living daylights out of you, but when you see it you can't stop laughing.

It's the same with porn. We all have our own sensibilities and perceptions, so an adult film that seems totally exciting to one person may bore somebody else to tears, or a film that impresses someone as delicate and refined may strike you as over the top and depraved.

Human sexuality is very diverse, and that is what's so great about not just life but also pornographic films. To each his or her own. Some people derive sexual pleasure from a pie in the face, some are crazy about latex, and some are foot or shoe fetishists. Others are attracted to men, and

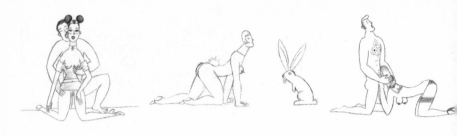

still others are drawn to women or cross-dressers or transpeople. There are butt freaks and people who are into heavy S&M, people who dream of romantic lovemaking in front of a fire and people who want rough anonymous sex in public places, people who like being tied up and people who enjoy the torture of being tickled with feathers. With six billion people in the world, there are six billion ways to get off.

Information is what matters here, just the way it does in other areas of your life. The more you know about sex, the more opportunities you have to make choices, and the more you can explore and enjoy your sexuality.

In any case, modern women and men are allowed to indulge their fantasies, and that means sampling a few flavors off the beaten path of sexual tastes. Chocolate may be your favorite, but every now and then you can try something else for a change, even if all you end up doing is confirming your preference for chocolate. In sex as in food, variety is the spice of life, and from time to time you may be in the mood for something different.

When I bring this topic up with my women friends, many of them admit having tastes in porn that aren't necessarily related to what they usually do in bed. Adult films let them take a realistic, very graphic peek at sexual practices they may not be brave enough (or interested enough) to try on their own. I've found myself among women who

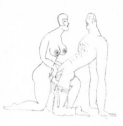 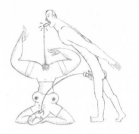 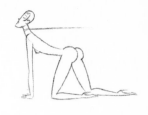

enjoy watching sex between two good-looking gay men, women who fantasize about bisexuality and want to see two women together or feel like stealing a quick glance at the world of S&M or fetishism. I've talked with punked-out girls who just love to watch ultra-Barbies like Jenna Jameson in action, demure preppies who enjoy Belladonna's brand of rough, perverted porn, and women who fantasize about being overpowered by a total stranger or having sex in public.

And you can enjoy every one of these adventures safely and comfortably on your TV or computer screen, without having to interact with anyone else or put yourself in risky situations. Aren't adult films fantastic?

Information leads to freedom of choice, and freedom leads to pleasure. You can't say you don't like adult films if you've never watched so much as a single pornographic scene. That's like saying you don't like oysters if you've never tried them (they're delicious, as a matter of fact, especially with a little lemon and pepper and some finely chopped red onion on top).

THE WISE WANKER

There's a new girl in town—the wise wanker. She doesn't need anyone to cater to her sexual whims. She pursues pleasure without guilt, and she knows and respects her own body. She knows how to enjoy sex with herself, she has sexual smarts and emotional intelligence, and she knows where to look for sex toys. She knows what she wants, and she knows how to get it.

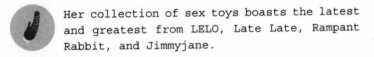 She knows that the Internet is rich with possibilities, and she knows how to make the most of it. She reads sex blogs written by other women and maybe even writes one of her own. She knows all about the new adult boutiques and sex toys, she watches adult movies online, and she looks for lovers—and finds them, too.

Her collection of sex toys boasts the latest and greatest from LELO, Late Late, Rampant Rabbit, and Jimmyjane.

In her DVD collection you'll find movies like *Shortbus*, *9 Songs*, *Five Hot Stories for Her*, *Behind the Green Door*, *Secretary*, and *Faster, Pussycat! Kill! Kill!* The wise wanker knows her porn, and she's researched all kinds to discover her tastes.

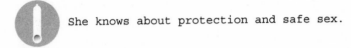 She knows about protection and safe sex.

Her library includes books by Anaïs Nin, Marguerite Duras, Virginie Despentes, Linda Williams, Catherine Millet, Colette, and Pauline Réage.

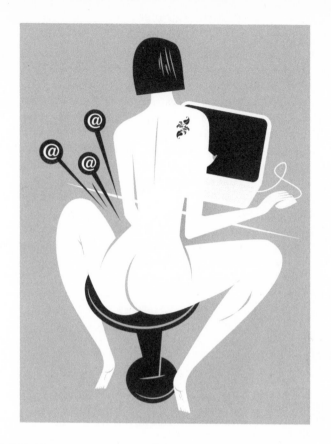

CAUTION: SEX UP AHEAD

What's up with the sex in mainstream Hollywood
movies? They treat sex so badly that they've
spawned a flourishing multimillion-dollar industry of sexually explicit, X-rated, pornographic
movies—films for grownups, you might say, movies
made for adult men and women.

Sex usually comes in for disparaging treatment
at the hands of mainstream filmmakers. It's as if
they're saying, "This is *serious cinema*. If you
want porn, go rent yourself an X-rated movie."
But sexuality is actually one of a human being's
most defining characteristics, often so central

to a person's life that it can't be isolated and concealed for the sake of telling a story.

In literature, sex is out in the open, not hidden away. But the film industry has always been hypocritical, fearful, and puritanical when it comes to putting sex on the screen.

Society has its rules to enforce, and even in our day and age the mass media are being used to impart moral instruction and perpetuate the ideal of the "respectable" woman. But I'm sick and tired of what I call the "whorifying" of women—the act of calling women whores if they enjoy guilt-free sex. This is something that happens all the time in mainstream movies.

SEX ON THE SCREEN

♀ Just when things start to get interesting, the camera cuts away, and the action instantly shifts to the following morning.

♀ If sex is shown in mainstream movies at all, it's treated like something dirty, dangerous, problematic, or sick.

♀ Mainstream movies are almost always made by men, and so an independent, sexually active, pleasure-seeking woman usually meets with disaster, almost always ending up raped, wounded, pregnant, or dead. Think of Sharon Stone in *Basic Instinct*, or Linda Fiorentino in *The Last Seduction*, or Meg Ryan in *In the Cut*.

♀ It's rare in a mainstream movie to find a woman who is both sexually active and happy.

Note: Part of the blame for the mishandling of sexuality in mainstream films lies with the Motion Picture Association of America's hypocritical, puritanical, conservative rating system. I highly recommend the excellent documentary *This Film Is Not Yet Rated*, Kirby Dick's fine exposé of how the rating system works.

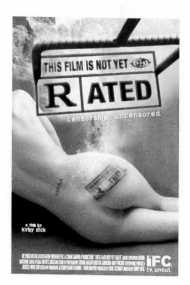

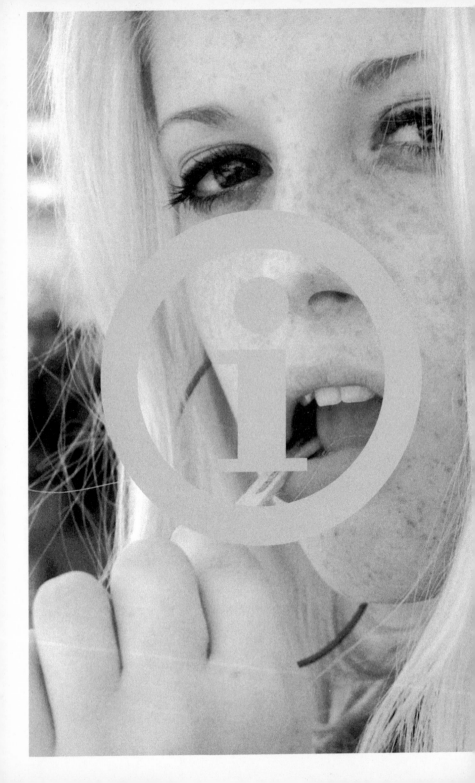

CHAPTER 7
A WORD TO THE WISE WANKER

Is there anything interesting out there for us? How do we sort through and enjoy all the different kinds of adult films? Mainstream porn and vintage erotic films, gay/lesbian/bisexual and fetish films, *hentai* and gonzo porn, do-it-yourself and New Wave porn, alt-porn—by the time you finish this chapter, you'll be an expert.

 RUSS MEYER

Boobs, Boobs, and More Boobs

One theory, which has its basis in pseudoscience, holds that men like big-breasted women because a woman like that is better equipped to nourish a man's future offspring. Another theory holds that men like big breasts because big breasts remind them of being nursed by their mothers. Still other theories have to do with being weaned too early or nursed too long (and with growing accustomed to having a breast nearby). If these theories hold water at all, more than one must have applied to Russ Meyer. How else to explain this legendary director's mammary fixation?

Russell Albion Meyer (1922–2004) was born in California to a policeman father and a mother who

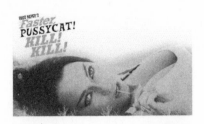
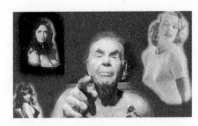
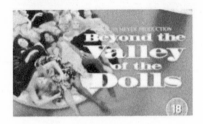
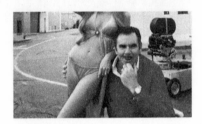
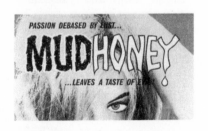
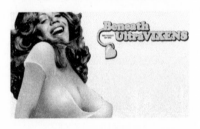
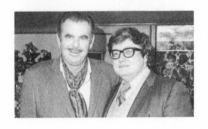
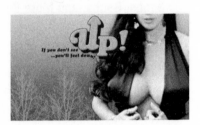

was a homemaker. He showed an interest in film at a very young age, and his mother supported her son's hobby by pawning her wedding ring to buy him an 8mm camera when he was only fourteen. With this camera, he shot several films that won prizes in local competitions, and he served as a U.S. Army combat cameraman during World War II. After the war, he went to work as a photographer for *Playboy*. During that period, he married a girl named Betty, but the marriage lasted less than a year.

Around the same time, he began directing "nudie-cutie" shorts. The first of these, *The French Peep Show* (1950), featured the burlesque star Tempest Storm. Nine years later, and now married to Eve Meyer, the actress and former *Playboy* Playmate of the Month, he directed *The Immoral Mr. Teas* (1959), his first commercially successful film and the first aboveground American movie to show nude female bodies without the excuse of naturalism, and with great respect for the female form in general and its anatomical beauty in particular. In this film, he also began to display a clear predilection for bringing humor into his movies, a touch that eventually became a hallmark of his work, as were his narrative techniques, which included numerous shots that lasted only five or ten seconds and gave his films a particular visual agility.

Then came the 1970s, and a series of movies (by now, their female stars' large breast size was a foregone conclusion) that began shaping the cinematic trend later known as sexploitation or grindhouse movies, a genre resembling softcore, which works nude or seminude women into the action whenever possible.

But the sweet taste of success wasn't Meyer's to savor until the release of *Faster, Pussycat! Kill! Kill!* (1965), a film that attained something approaching mainstream popularity. It can be considered a Z movie (the expression describes a low-budget production whose quirky charm makes it clearly different, if only for being bizarre). *Faster, Pussycat!* also launched an actress who was one of the director's favorites for a great part of her career—the sadistic and, of course, buxom Tura Satana. In this film she plays Varla, a go-go dancer who enjoys getting together with her co-workers Billie (Lori Williams) and Rosie (Haji) in their free time, when the three of them hit the road in their souped-up sports cars to look for trouble in the form of beatings, robberies, and murder. *Faster, Pussycat!* may be short on verisimilitude, but this film, like Russ Meyer's work in general, has been celebrated in feminist circles for its depiction of a woman who is powerful, independent, and strong, even though she's not exactly a saint.

Not long afterward came *Mondo Topless* (1966), Meyer's first color film. A "mockumentary" shot *cinéma vérité*-style, it portrays the lives of a group of San Francisco strippers. According to the film's publicity poster, "Russ Meyer's busty buxotic beauties" are "two much for one man!"

In 1968 came *Vixen*, another of the sagas that put Meyer on the map. The movie begins with the story of Vixen Palmer, a woman who lives in the Canadian Rockies. Her husband isn't around much, so she's forced to find new ways of entertaining herself. The film was such a success that 20th Century Fox offered Meyer a contract for his next three pictures.

The first of these was *Beyond the Valley of the Dolls* (1970), written by Meyer in collaboration with the film critic Roger Ebert, and purporting to be a sequel to *Valley of the Dolls* (1967), the film adaptation of Jacqueline Susann's 1966 novel. *Beyond the Valley of the Dolls* is a tale about three girls who want more than anything to break

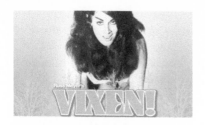

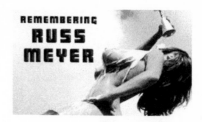

REMEMBERING
RUSS
MEYER

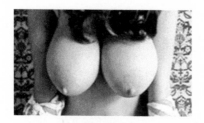

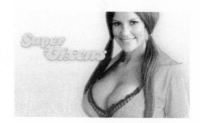

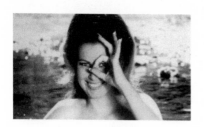

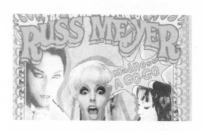

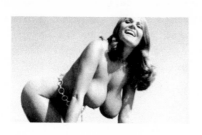

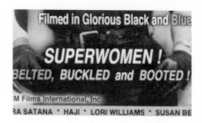

Filmed in Glorious Black and Blue

SUPERWOMEN !
BELTED, BUCKLED and BOOTED !

M Films International, Inc

RA SATANA * HAJI * LORI WILLIAMS * SUSAN BE

into show business. Susann's original story, filled with old-fashioned moralizing, gave Meyer and Ebert an opportunity to create a new version in which the three main characters, members of a rock band called The Kelly Affair, attempt to win at all costs in the city of Los Angeles and end up as alcoholic nymphomaniac drug addicts, victims of their own popularity. The film was released on the same day Meyer married a member of the film's cast, Edy Williams.

Supervixens (1975), Meyer's next successful feature, is a savage story about murder, sex, and violence in which a woman is not the executioner but the victim—a departure for Meyer. The following year, presumably to make up for *Supervixens*, Meyer directed *Up!* (1976), whose protagonist, Adolf, bears a certain resemblance to another, more famous Adolf and surrenders to all sorts of masochistic sexual practices, only to be devoured in the end by the piranha that a criminal hand has slipped into his bathtub.

The last film Meyer released before a filmmaking hiatus of more than twenty years was *Beneath the Valley of the Ultra-Vixens* (1979), which portrays the adventures of Lamar, a man who decides to throw himself at every woman he meets so he can discover the cause of his problem—his inability to satisfy Lavonia, his voluptuous wife. This is regarded as one of the director's most outrageous films, and its peculiar dark humor makes it strong stuff even for the director's most loyal fans.

After *Beneath the Valley of the Ultra-Vixens*, which happened to coincide with the start of the silicone-implant trend among actresses, Meyer stopped making movies until 2001, when he released *Pandora Peaks*, in which the stripper who gives the film its name performs one routine after another, to her own and the director's voice-overs.

94

On September 18, 2004, Russ Meyer died of pneumonia at the age of eighty-two. It was reported that he had been suffering from advanced senile dementia for years, and that his body was too weak to resist the infection. I think that this lover of natural female beauty may have been fed up with so many silicone breasts, and that his body said, "Enough," perhaps to give him, in death, the same sensually tinged air of Greek tragedy that informs his movies.

Let's hope he's resting in peace, wherever he is, surrounded by nymphs who are busty and eternally topless, the way he liked to show them.

BLAXPLOITATION

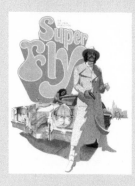

Russ Meyer's work was a precursor of sexploitation, a genre that was immediately followed in the United States by blaxploitation movies. This genre featured African American actors in productions that mixed the funk music of the era with street fighting, stories about sex and drugs and mules, and spectacular, scantily clad females. In the 1970s, African Americans were continuing to demand their civil rights as well as their right to be represented in art and culture, including the movies. *Superfly*, with music by Curtis Mayfield, and the legendary *Shaft*, with a sound track by Isaac Hayes, are two good examples of a genre that enjoyed a major revival several years ago, thanks in large part to Quentin Tarantino, a great fan of blaxploitation films.

THE 1970S

Porn as Cult Film, Art, and Experimentation

From a woman's point of view, or from the point of view of anyone who hoped to find something more in adult films than coarse scenes of penetration and crude medical shots, the best time for pornographic movies was certainly the 1970s. That was when a number of directors were endowing their films with intelligent dialogue, interesting plots, and sometimes even social and satirical content. In the United States, with personal possession of pornography having been decriminalized in 1969,[1] porn managed for the first time to break out of the limited world of grindhouse theaters, and it became a cult phenomenon on the spot, without having to wait years for validation from some gaggle of film freaks.

Mona: The Virgin Nymph (1970), a fifty-nine-minute film produced by Bill Osco and directed by Michael Benveniste and Howard Ziehm, is regarded as the first pornographic movie with an actual plot to have opened in American theaters. In *Mona*, a young woman (Fifi Watson) is initiated into oral sex by her father, whose intention (pure-minded, of course) is to preserve his daughter's virginity for her wedding night. Mona then proceeds to exercise her oral skills on every man she meets. The film cost $7,000 to make and took in more than $2 million—the shot heard 'round the world for high-quality porn.

All of this was partly due to the sexual freedom that had been in the air since the late 1960s, in the United States as well as in Europe. Thanks to the Pill, and to the (relative) availability and acceptability of abortion, sex was taken off the roster of mortal sins, and the concept of free love appeared along with porn chic. Porn chic was born in the early 1970s with movies like *Flesh Gordon* (1974), a blockbuster with special effects

96

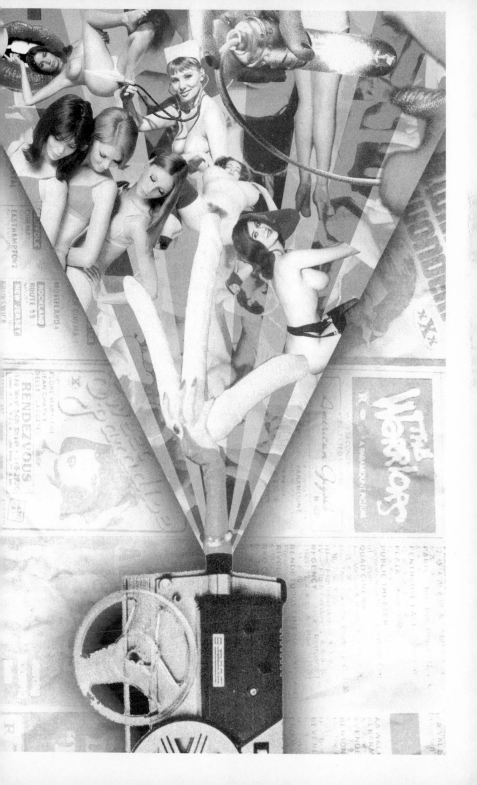

and makeup by the renowned Rick Baker. Another influential film was *Boys in the Sand* (1971), the first gay porn film to achieve crossover success. It was also the first porn film to include credits for its cast and crew, the first to parody the title of a mainstream stage play and film (Mart Crowley's *Boys in the Band*), and the first to be reviewed in the *New York Times*. Porn chic also enjoyed a vogue in Europe, where the term referred to movies like *Emmanuelle*—the white Emmanuelle, the black Emmanuelle, the Emmanuelle in outer space, and any of the other Emmanuelles in more than thirty sequels that were made of that film.

From that point on, the names of directors like Gerard Damiano (undoubtedly the most important figure from porn's golden age), Radley Metzger (who also went by the pseudonym Henry Paris), and Sharon McNight (the first woman to direct an adult film, *The Autobiography of a Flea*, produced by the Mitchell Brothers in 1976) were on everyone's lips. They were not regarded as B movie directors (or even Z movie directors, as they would be today) but were treated like legitimate celebrities on TV, at film festivals, and elsewhere.

Gerard Damiano deserves special mention. His films were a far cry from today's porn with its perfect, huge-breasted women. He even replaced the nineteen-year-old unknown actress who was going to star in *The Devil in Miss Jones* with the already mature Georgina Spelvin so he could give the role more character. How many directors today would switch from their flavor-of-the-month bimbo to a mother of two for the sake of making a more realistic movie? After that came *The Story of Joanna* (a masochistic fantasy based on *The Story of O*) and *Memories Within Miss Aggie*, about an old woman in a dark room recounting her sexual experiences to a mystery man whose face we never see. The latter film, so depressing that it inspired more jeers than cheers, was quickly pulled from many adult theaters.

And then there were the Mitchell Brothers, Artie and Jim, with their hippie porn (so called because of its psychedelic images and its sound tracks supplied by West Coast rock bands). Their work marked an era that began with *Behind the Green Door* and came to an end in the early 1990s, when Artie Mitchell, his alcoholism and cocaine use said to be out of control, died at the hands of his brother, who shot him point-blank with a .22 rifle. Performers at the Mitchell Brothers' O'Farrell Theatre, the strip club founded by the brothers and still in operation, bade farewell to Artie with a huge wild party that went on for more than three days.[2]

But none of this would have been possible without the real stars—the actors and actresses who lent their faces (and bodies) to all these terrific productions. They ranged from the divine Marilyn Chambers, the Ivory Snow girl who became half the planet's wet dream, to the throaty Linda Lovelace and Georgina Spelvin—and let's not forget the prodigious John Holmes (the adult film industry's first AIDS casualty, sad to say).

Many people, blown away by the quality of golden age porn, had been thinking the same thing that the writer and director William Rotsler said in 1973: "Erotic films are here to stay. Eventually they will simply merge into the mainstream of motion pictures and disappear as a labeled sub-division. Nothing can stop this."[3]

He was wrong, of course. The 1980s—the decade of what were, broadly speaking, the tackiest fashions ever—managed to give us fluorescent colors, shoulder pads, leg warmers, and much more. Porn chic is dead; long live porn chic!

FIVE WAYS TO TELL YOU'RE WATCHING 1970S PORN

1. The female star's untrimmed, unwaxed pubic hair

2. The absence of silicone-enhanced lips, breasts, and cheekbones

3. Your continued interest, even after you've come, in seeing how the story turns out

4. The dimensions and cut of the underwear

5. Dialogue that goes beyond "I'm here to repair your pipes"

THE TOP TEN FILMS OF PORN'S GOLDEN AGE

Deep Throat (1972)

Behind the Green Door (1972)

The Devil in Miss Jones (1973)

Insatiable (1980)

The Opening of Misty Beethoven (1976)

The Resurrection of Eve (1973)

The Story of Joanna (1975)

Flesh Gordon (1974)

Sodom and Gomorrah: The Last Seven Days (1975)

Sexorcist Devil (1974)

MAINSTREAM PORN

The Business of Churning Out Movies

The phrase *mainstream porn* refers to the porn that began to appear in the 1980s, when VCRs came on the market. In other words, it's the kind of porn that most people (especially men) are watching these days, the kind in which the men are virile, muscled, and well hung and all the women are potentially bisexual, perpetually astonished to discover a penis inside a pair of boxers, and willing to have sex with the first guy who happens by. The actresses in mainstream porn are usually thin, too, with big boobs and full lips (sometimes too full), and they feel no qualms about shrieking when they have an orgasm. They enjoy taking a load of cum in the face, and they don't seem to mind when it gets in their eyes (that alone is almost enough to make them sexual superheroines).

A few mainstream porn actors and actresses, and even some directors of mainstream porn, have broken out to become household names, sometimes after working in other kinds of films (Rocco Siffredi appeared in *Romance*, for example, and Traci Lords doesn't do porn at all anymore), or recording a pop song, or sometimes when their life stories became material for a biopic, as happened with the unfortunately famous John Holmes and the movie *Boogie Nights*.

A mainstream porn production can cost anywhere from around $10,000 for a low-budget film intended for a late-late-night TV audience (these productions are churned out like sausages, in terms of both speed and, unfortunately, quality) to $1 million, which is what it cost to make the movie said to be the most expensive X-rated film ever—*Pirates*, produced by Digital Playground and Adam & Eve. *Pirates*, inspired by the Hollywood blockbuster

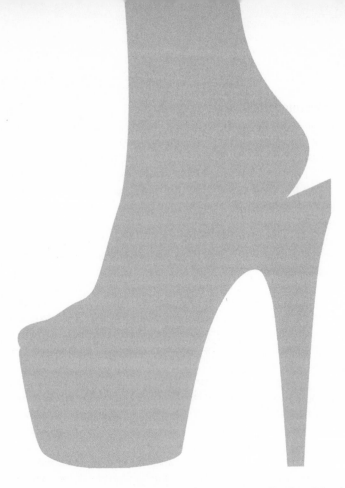

Pirates of the Caribbean: The Curse of the Black Pearl, was directed by the award-winning Joone. It stars performers like Jesse Jane, Carmen Luvana, Devon, and Jenaveve Jolie, and its scenery and costumes are of unusually high quality for porn.

Mainstream pornographic films also have a fairly rigid structure because they have to be morally acceptable (believe it or not, there are things in porn that are morally unacceptable, especially in the United States, for example), which means they run the risk of becoming repetitive and therefore boring. In short, the only acceptable sex acts in this kind of porn are those that a moderately liberated couple might try in bed at home. They range from fellatio to cunnilingus to masturbation to coitus to ejaculation on the girl's face—lather, rinse, repeat. Never, ever, under any circumstances, needless to say, will a man touch, kiss, or penetrate another man, and the male actors in scenes featuring threesomes are famously careful to avoid even brushing up against each other. Throw in the women characters' bisexuality and their complete willingness to jump into a threesome, and there you have it—the basic structure of a movie that can be summed up in a few phrases like "BLONDE blows BLACK GUY," "REDHEAD goes down on BLONDE," and "BLACK GUY mounts REDHEAD from behind." Once in a while a screenplay may add something else, but that's not always necessary, and even when it is, the additional material usually could have been written by a chimp.

A typical device in this kind of production is to create a pornographic version of a blockbuster classic, turning *Star Trek: The Next Generation* into *Sex Trek: The Next Penetration*, or making *The Terminator* into *The Penetrator* and *Titanic* into *Tittanic* (with a DVD cover showing a priceless image of the ship with two gigantic boobs, one at port and the other at starboard), or remaking *The Blair Witch Project*, all too predictably, as *The Blair Bitch Project*. These titles look like something dreamed up by bored teenage boys playing a game, but a look around the Internet will convince you they're as real as can be.

Now that we know what mainstream porn is all about, doesn't it make you feel like demanding a new kind of porn? It's too bad that the adult film industry is pushing such a pathetic, heterocentric view of sex, and that adolescents are soaking it up as if it were actual sex education. Revolution now!

SOME MAJOR PORN PRODUCTION COMPANIES

Beate Uhse	Ninn Worx
Club Jenna	Penthouse
Colmax	Playboy
Daring!	Private Media Group
Digital Playground	Red Light District
Elegant Angel	Spice Studios
Productions	Teravision
Evil Angel	Vivid Entertainment
Hustler	Wicked Pictures
Marc Dorcel	Woodman Entertainment
Mercenary Pictures	Zero Tolerance

 GONZO

It Doesn't Get Any Cheaper Than This

At one time or another you must have heard the word *gonzo,* and not just in reference to adult films. The term was originally used to describe the writings of Hunter S. Thompson, author of the famous *Fear and Loathing in Las Vegas*, a book of reportage that Terry Gilliam brilliantly adapted for the screen in 1998. Thompson, an intrepid journalist who took to writing his pieces by becoming a participant-observer, ended up including himself as one more figure taking part in the stories he was reporting.

As an extrapolation of this concept, gonzo porn is a genre in which the director also participates, by giving instructions to the actors and actresses or even by appearing in the shot himself (sometimes the camera is shown, too). As a rule, gonzo porn is completely devoid of plot elements, and much of it uses the convention of the casting couch (interviews with aspiring actresses) or "girl on the street" interviews. Either way, the girl undresses as the interview goes on, until she's having unvarnished hardcore sex. The main reason for posing direct questions to the performers is to get the audience involved more as participants than as spectators.

Films in this genre tend to last precisely ninety minutes and consist of several scenes, each fifteen to thirty minutes long, in which the lead actor—female or male (low-budget films are among the most democratic, so gonzo is also a gay genre)—masturbates or has sex with one or more partners. The scenes, once shot, are not cut or edited (most of the time, anyway), and so they can seem extremely long, even boring. Gonzo doesn't require any advance work, since there is no screenplay (although certain questions do always seem to be asked—really imaginative ones like "How old were you when you lost your virginity?" and "Do you like big cocks?"), and gonzo also doesn't need much in terms of production, since most gonzo movies are shot in hotels, more or less cheap ones, with a handheld or tripod-mounted video camera. There is also no need for costumes, makeup, or hair styling, so gonzo films don't cost much to make. The gonzo genre became very fashionable in the late 1980s and reached its peak in the late 1990s.

 CANDIDA ROYALLE

The First Women's Porn
It took us a while, but—steadily, little by little—we came to see that traditional porn was for men, and that for women there was no porn at all (much less feminist porn). Candida Royalle is clearly a pioneer in the area of adult movies written and directed from a woman's point of view, and she was the first to see women as a potential audience for X-rated films.

In the beginning, woman-oriented films weren't even characterized as porn for women. They were characterized as erotica for couples, and their purpose was basically educational—to make things easier for women who, for cultural and personal reasons, were having trouble talking openly about what they needed in bed, and to light a fire under longtime couples as well as those who had fallen into a rut and lost their passion or their desire to try new things. In fact, Candida Royalle's films are widely used by American sex therapists who work with couples.

As a director, Candida Royalle tried from the start to give her films the touch of sweetness and tenderness she thought was missing from pornographic movies, and she added other elements meant to make her films more woman-friendly. She began her professional porn career after moving to San Francisco from her hometown, New York, in search of a more open lifestyle. In San Francisco she devoted herself to making art, performing in avant-garde theater, and singing in jazz clubs. She was looking for extra work as an artist's model when an agent asked her if she wanted to act in a pornographic movie. "I was really insulted," she says. "I had never even seen one, and I stormed out of his office." But her boyfriend at the time was offered the lead in Anthony Spinelli's film *Cry for Cindy* (1976). "I got to see what it was like by visiting the set of his movie," Royalle says. "And I realized this is not the sleazy environment that I thought it was, it was very professional. The money was good for a struggling artist, cultural attitudes toward sex at that time were quite open, and back then there were no serious life-threatening diseases" such as AIDS.[4]

Her extensive acting career (she appeared in some seventy films), together with the need to make porn that was a better fit with her ethical and aesthetic values, then led her to become a director. The last film she starred in, which she also wrote and directed, was *Blue Magic* (1980), four years before founding her own company, Femme Productions. Today the company has a division called Femme Chocolat, which produces ethnically diverse erotica featuring African American performers. Over time, Candida Royalle has proved to be a successful businesswoman and has created her own line of sex toys, among other products.

SEVEN THINGS THAT MAKE CANDIDA ROYALLE'S MOVIES DIFFERENT

1. The women portrayed in her films are educated, intelligent, and able to think for themselves. There are no Lolitas being seduced by lustful professors, and no housewives jumping into bed with the plumber.

2. Silicone is either glaringly absent or very discreet. The women look more like the girl next door than traditional porn bimbos.

3. The men are more attractive and, within the limits of the business, better mannered. For the Royalle women, there are no hairy little trolls like Ron Jeremy shouting "Suck me, bitch!"

4. A scene doesn't end right after the man comes. There are kisses afterward, along with caresses and even promises of eternal love—more or less the way things are in real life.

5. Blow jobs don't last for hours, and they're usually the reward for a long, diligent session of cunnilingus.

(continued on page 108)

(continued from page 107)

6. The women are able to have and express reservations. They can say "Not here" or "Not now" (although the truth is that they never take long to change their minds), and they can complain because a partner, in a fit of passion, is tearing the elastic on their favorite underwear.

7. The dialogue is somewhat more elaborate, and the films have a plot, or at least they make an effort, since that, after all, is what it's all about.

CANDIDA ROYALLE: FILMOGRAPHY

Femme (1984)

Urban Heat (1984)

Three Daughters (1986)

Christine's Secret (1986)

A Taste of Ambrosia (1987)

Rites of Passion (1987)

Sensual Escape (1988)

Revelations (1993)

My Surrender (1996)

The Gift (1997)

The Bridal Shower (1997)

One Size Fits All (1998)

Eyes of Desire (1998)

Eyes of Desire 2 (1999)

Under the Covers (2007)

REALITY PORN

Bogus Reality Sells

It's nighttime, and we're on a beach that's all but deserted. Barcelona, Cancún, Playa de Aro, Ipanema—it's always the same. The quality of the grainy images is so poor that we wouldn't be able to make out the palm trees even if there were any. In fact, this film appears to have been shot with a cell phone. All of a sudden a cute couple enters the picture. These two have been drinking—or, if not, they're in a very good mood. They fling themselves onto the sand, in what little shelter a few deck chairs can provide, and begin to kiss. Things heat up, and they take off their clothes (or just tug articles of clothing up or down, depending) and start making love. They switch positions, nibbling and licking and fondling breasts and nipples, often completely oblivious to the astonished passersby staring at them. And suddenly they're done. They put their clothes back on (or back in place) and sit gazing at the moon, or they go back to wherever they came from, and nobody bats an eye. These seaside trysts can also occur in a car, in a park, or in the restroom at a dance club (to each his own). In a word, what we've known forever as the "quickie" has now become a cheap, potent subgenre of pornography.

Which brings us to reality porn, an adult film genre with plenty of fans, since audiences are taken in by the pretense of watching real sex rather than actors in staged scenes. But there's a reason why every law, as they say, has its loophole—this kind of film is legally very dubious, and it's very easy to sue if a film can be traced back to its creator, and so professional or aspiring actors and actresses are usually hired to appear in what the tabloid press likes to call "candid"

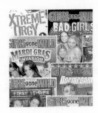
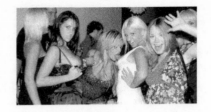

videos (though there's almost nothing candid about them), and that's that—no harm, no foul. As a minor genre, reality porn doesn't have much of a presence in the DVD market, so this kind of film is primarily sold and viewed on the Internet. One of the most famous examples of the genre is the *Girls Gone Wild* series (www.girlsgonewild.com), in which the filmmakers hang around youth hot spots (such as New Orleans during Mardi Gras, or other locations that college students favor for spring break) looking for attractive girls who have had too much to drink and are willing to take their clothes off in exchange for a T-shirt featuring the Girls Gone Wild logo. Basically, these films show breasts, butts, and genitals, but sometimes the girls are followed back to their hotel rooms or to particular gathering spots where they are urged to have sex with each other. The reality porn industry, always pushing the limits, has had a number of run-ins with the authorities and has also been hit with some civil lawsuits. But, thanks to legal loopholes, the defendants have usually managed to get their way, and otherwise they've been slapped with fines in various amounts, which they've paid without a peep—apparently all those girls going wild are earning them more than enough to cover that particular expense.

Videos and photographs of ex-girlfriends are another hot Internet commodity, and that's really too bad, since making films and taking pictures can be an important element of sex play but can also end

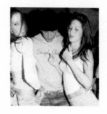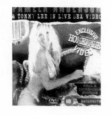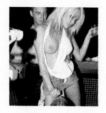

up being used against you when you least expect it. Breaking up is already hard enough to do, without surfing the web later on and coming face to face with your own butt.

Still another popular type of reality porn displays famous women caught going commando, that is, without underwear—Britney Spears and Paris Hilton are a couple of real experts on this genre—or flashing a nipple while topless at the beach, or striking a sexy pose. And the star prize within this genre is reality porn that catches someone having full-out sex. Ever since Italian magazines published more than forty photos of Daniel Ducruet, then the husband of Princess Stephanie of Monaco, enjoying a naked poolside romp with a Belgian stripper named Fili Houteman (a video was released, too, but was soon confiscated), it's been open season on leaked celebrity sex. Some time after the Ducruet affair, two of the world's most famous bottle blondes, Paris Hilton and Pamela Anderson, somehow made the mistake of allowing their hottest sex videos to be leaked on the Internet and released as DVDs.

Another curious example of bogus reality on the Internet is the Bang Bus website (www.bangbus.com), an online business founded by Kristopher Hinson and Penn Davis, two misogynist buddies who met at the University of Florida. Each Bang Bus video features a girl who is picked up on the street and persuaded to enter a van that is completely outfitted for sex. The girl is then filmed having sex with several men in the back of the van, and even with the camera itself, while the van is in motion. Afterward she's usually cheated out of the money she was promised and is dropped off naked at some random spot along the highway, far from home, at which point the van takes off, with the driver and the cameraman laughing. Hinson and Davis are a couple of hustlers who have made millions staging the same scene hundreds of times.

SEX, HOLLYWOOD STYLE

Puritanism Versus Business

The line between eroticism and pornography is a fine one and easy to cross, and the old saying that suggesting is better than showing (a saying well known to movie stars of the 1950s) has been burned into the mind of many a director. As a result, quite a few Hollywood movies, without being X-rated or even softcore films, are memorable for their sexy, bold, clearly suggestive images.

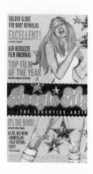 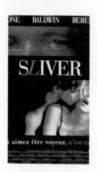 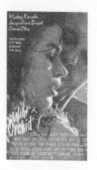 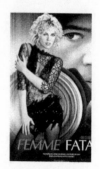

Consider *9½ Weeks*, for example. What do you remember about that movie? Probably not the dialogue, or the names of the producer and the director, but Kim Basinger gyrating to Joe Cocker's "You Can Leave Your Hat On," or maybe the scene where Mickey Rourke (before he turned into the elephant he is today) cooks her dinner, making such an impression that he himself ends up as dessert.

We've known for a long time that sex in the media sells. Just turn on the TV if you want to see naked (or half naked) women in commercials for shampoo, cars, deodorants, and perfumes. If there's a long leg or the hint of a breast or belly button on the screen, that's where people are going to focus. And once an advertiser has their attention, bingo! They're his.

Unfortunately, the way directors use this power to spark the erotic imagination is completely up to them. One director may use it for product enhancement in a teen sex comedy, as when Shannon Elizabeth is spied on through a webcam while performing a striptease in *American Pie*. Another director may use it to recoup the millions he's paying some sex symbol (or maybe you thought Bo Derek was half naked in all those movies because of the heat).

Speaking of stripping, Jane Fonda, star of the psychedelically inflected *Barbarella* (1968),

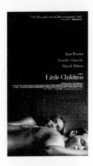 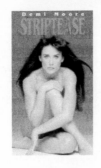 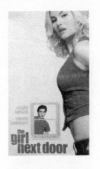 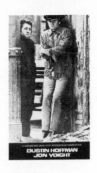

surely one of the most artistic films of all time, takes off her space suit (designed by Paco Rabanne, of course) to sensuous music in conditions of zero gravity, and throughout the movie she devotes her powers of seduction, which lead her into situations that include a lesbian dalliance with Anita Pallenberg, to saving Dr. Durand Durand, the mad scientist.

Not surprisingly, another movie with a leitmotif of stripping is *Striptease* (1996), in which Demi Moore plays a single mother who dances to earn money for a child custody fight but gets into serious trouble when a congressman (Burt Reynolds) becomes infatuated with her. The film, roundly panned by critics, was a big hit with audiences, which just goes to show that this wasn't the worst way to see Demi Moore naked. In the same vein, Elizabeth Berkley in Paul Verhoeven's *Showgirls* (1995) portrays Naomi Malone, a young woman all set to become the top showgirl in Las Vegas, but not without first violating her own ethical code.

As we've seen, another moneymaking move is suggestiveness. But tell that to Sharon Stone, who has been the owner of Hollywood's most popular pubis ever since she brought the mysterious Catherine Tramell to life in *Basic Instinct* (1992). (Stone never actually did expose herself, no matter how many people all over the world, remote control in hand, have drained millions of batteries trying to prove that she did.) Catherine is the whole nine yards—in addition to dropping hints about her involvement in a love triangle, she cavorts with a pre-Botox Michael Douglas, dances dirty with another girl in a disco, and enjoys playing with ice picks. Another actress who excels in playing a cold, ruthless seductress is Rebecca Romijn-Stamos in *Femme Fatale* (2002), who certainly did get naked (but showed very little) to play the mysterious wife of the American ambassador to Paris. Two actresses who will go down (so to speak) in history for one hot scene are Susan Sarandon and Catherine Deneuve in *The Hunger* (1983) as they get caught up in an aesthetically sinister lesbian adventure that will make your hair stand on end, though not exactly from fear; never has there been a more mouthwatering vampire than Deneuve, as seen through the lens of Tony Scott. And Neve Campbell and Denise Richards are no slouches, either, playing the evil Suzie Toller and Kelly Van Ryan in *Wild Things* (1998), in which they ruin the life of a high school guidance counselor played by Matt Dillon. Anyone who has seen this movie will remember the two of them kissing in the pool, a scene so hot and heavy that the water looks as if it might come to a boil.

Finally, two films that exude sensuality from the first frame to the last are Stanley Kubrick's *Eyes Wide Shut* (1999), in which Tom Cruise and Nicole Kidman, as Bill and Alice Harford, are introduced to the world of upper-class private orgies, and *The Postman Always Rings Twice* (1981), the remake of Tay Garnett's 1946 classic, although this time director Bob Rafelson highlights what has to be the most sexually charged role in film history, thanks in large part to David Mamet's adapted screenplay. One thing is for sure—no one who sees this film will ever be able to look at a kitchen table the same way again.

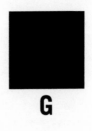

G

L

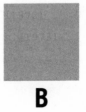

B

T

116

GAY, LESBIAN, BISEXUAL, TRANSGENDER: GLBT

In Sex and Porn, There's No Accounting for Taste

The gay community has spent years putting its stamp on all kinds of things. There's a whole society of gay consumers with their own music, their own divas, and even their own hotels and travel agencies. Decades of coming out have left very few gay men and lesbian women still living in the closet.

For the most part, gay men have an unconflicted, "anything goes" attitude toward their sexuality, since their liberation is fairly recent and is still evolving. This is not to say that gay men are promiscuous, but only that after waging a tough battle against others' prejudices, they're finally enjoying their hard-won freedom to do as they please with their own bodies. As a result, there's a big market for gay porn, and it's reflected in the existence of specialized porn producers, dedicated TV channels, gay porn film festivals, and large amounts of amateur gay porn on the Internet. Men who like both men and porn need a market of their own, and we've already seen why—it's because men in traditional porn never, ever touch, since that would be considered a grave offense against masculinity. And if they don't touch, forget about them kissing, jerking each other off, or penetrating each other, acts seen only in queer porn. Films made from a bisexual point of view are harder to find, although indie porn is doing a lot to make bi films a respectable genre. A standout in this category is *The Bi Apple*, a film by the New York director Audacia Ray.

In 1971, *Boys in the Sand* was released, and it was the first gay film to be recognized as such— although you didn't have to try very hard to find patently gay content in the videos that Andy Warhol, Kenneth Anger, and Paul Morrissey were making in the late 1960s. Things have changed a lot since then, and I'm not just talking about things like bell-bottoms. To begin with, a number of women decided to claim queer porn for their own use—if you can get turned on by one good-looking guy (and, yes, the gay audience usually does care about good looks), then why wouldn't you get turned on watching two good-looking guys kissing and making love? And even lesbians and bisexuals say they like *yaoi manga*, in which the protagonists are effeminate men. If we add this group of women viewers to all the men watching gay porn, we can understand why production companies like Lucas Entertainment, Eurocream, and Cazzo Film (which counts the cult director Bruce LaBruce among its collaborators) are doing so well and making films with bigger and bigger budgets. One Spanish production company worth mentioning is Jalif Studio, where the director Jalif is reinventing gay porn with his fresh ideas and modern outlook.

These days there's a raging debate, as well as serious division in the industry, over bareback sex (that is, sex without condoms or other protection), a practice at some studios despite opposition from the big production companies, which see these studios as putting porn in a bad light and contributing to the spread of HIV. Another interesting feature of gay porn is that it includes a large number of subgenres for fetishists whose tastes range from guys dressed in military or other types of uniforms to guys in athletic attire like tracksuits or white tennis shorts.

The past few years have seen a boom in transgender porn, and to exploit this new niche even traditional porn stars like Nacho Vidal have started their own production companies (Vidal's is in Brazil), although their movies are usually pretty simpleminded and treat transgender people more like circus freaks than like feeling, sexually complex people. But several promising new directors, such as Morty Diamond, are offering a newer and more authentic point of view (Diamond's documentary about a transgender couple, *Trans Entities: The Nasty Love of Papí and Wil*, is discussed later in this chapter, in the section titled "Documentaries"). Also worth mentioning are the films of Buck Angel, especially *Couch Surfers*, from Trannywood Pictures (www.trannywoodpictures.com).

And what about the girls? Like the song says, they just want to have fun, and in the battle for a new lesbian porn they're fighting like regular Amazons. It may not be true that every single traditional pornographic film contains a lesbian scene, but 99 percent of them certainly do (the exception is Japanese porn, where lesbian scenes occur only in films of the *rezu* genre). But one lesbian scene isn't enough to turn a movie into a lesbian film, of course, especially since a man can show up at any point to crash the party and get a blow job à deux. Traditional porn may offer lesbians a few tidbits, but it can also leave them feeling deeply offended by the remaining scenes, in which women become mere objects to be handled by a domineering male.

As a result, lesbians decided to take the bull by the horns and launch their own porn revolution, one that took shape primarily in film schools and art schools, the breeding grounds for such movement leaders as Shine Louise Houston, Nan Kinney (founder of the Fatale Media production company and co-founder of the magazine *On Our Backs*, two absolute touchstones of dyke porn), Angie Dowling, and the sophisticated Maria Beatty. All these directors show actual sex between women who do not have long nails, are not constantly looking at the camera, and are not waiting for some guy to join them in bed so the "real" sex can begin. Another authentic lesbian pornographer is the Canadian director Bren Ryder, who runs the very successful Good Dyke Porn production company (www.gooddykeporn.com).

BONDAGE, FETISHISM, AND S&M

Whips, Pinups, Impossibly High Heels, Latex, and Submission in the New Porn

And now we come to the fantastic world of bondage, fetishism, and sadomasochism, three highly aesthetic, richly nuanced forms of sexuality that have gone off the porn reservation and burst into scenes and films that have earned their place in the collective erotic imagination. Who hasn't seen *Belle de Jour*, the Luis Buñuel film in which Catherine Deneuve plays a middle-class housewife whose masochistic impulses lead her into prostitution? Is there anyone who's left cold by the ultrasexy pinup girl Bettie Page and her playmate, Tempest Storm? Is there anyone who missed *In the Realm of the Senses*, the X-rated Japanese film screened at Cannes in 1976? And what about that scene in *The Graduate* where Dustin Hoffman catches sight of Anne Bancroft's provocatively extended leg and unshod foot? All of this, and much more, is bondage, fetishism, and S&M as found in the movies.

But let's take a closer look at these phenomena so their fine points won't escape us. Bondage is physical restraint—using special ropes, chains (although chains would actually bring this practice closer to S&M), and often gags—involving all or part of an erotic partner's clothed or nude body. Bondage may be used as an aesthetic-erotic practice, as one element of a sadomasochistic relationship, or as part of a domination ritual. There are very strict safety rules that every practitioner is expected to know (for example, no one is ever tied up and left alone, and a rope is never tied around the neck). Fetishism (the word is derived from Latin *facticius*, meaning "artificial") is a paraphilia in which an individual becomes aroused or reaches orgasm by means of a talisman or fetish, which can be anything

120

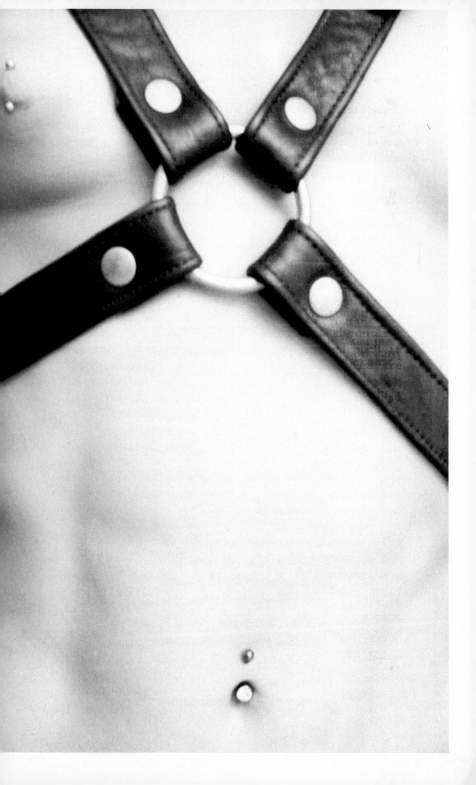

from an object to a substance to a smell to a part of the body. It is not regarded as pathological as long as it doesn't provoke clinical symptoms in the practitioner or in his or her partners. Vibrators, artificial vaginas, and other sex toys are not considered fetishes, since their actual purpose is sexual stimulation. And sadomasochism, as we saw in the glossary (chapter 5), takes its name from the surnames of the Marquis de Sade and Leopold von Sacher-Masoch, both of whose writings depict sexual relationships based on a dialectic of master and slave. In terms of modern sexuality, sadomasochism is a relationship between consenting adults who open themselves to the erotic possibilities of domination games, often without intercourse at all. Limits are negotiated beforehand, and the goal is mutual pleasure. There are no remaining copies of the first film to use BDSM content—*Am Sklavenmarkt* (*At the Slave Market*), directed sometime before 1910 by the Austrian filmmaker Johann Schwarzer—but the genre reached its peak in the 1970s, thanks largely to more or less free adaptations of Sade's work for the screen.

In the 1950s, Bettie Page acted in the best burlesque films, performed the most sensual stripteases, and posed for photographs that even today make her one of the best-known icons of fetishism and spanking. All the men's magazines of that era wanted her on their covers, and her collaboration with the photographer Bunny Yeager led to her appearance in the *Playboy* centerfold in January 1955, the same year Page was named Miss Pinup Girl of the World. Throughout her career she acted in short burlesque films like *Striporama*, *Varietease*, and *Teaserama* (mostly with Tempest Storm, her usual spankophile companion, who also appeared in several movies by Russ Meyer), and Page's work was later gathered into a single volume titled *The Bettie Page Collection*. Toward the end of the decade, Bettie Page got married, and not long afterward she experienced a religious conversion that prompted her to leave show business behind and disown her career as a sex symbol. From that point on, she worked for Christian organizations and wasn't heard from again.

In 1963, after the pinup era ended, Roger Vadim directed *Le Vice et la Vertu* (*Vice and Virtue*), with Robert Hossein and Catherine Deneuve, and cleared the way for the S&M movies of the 1970s. A few years later, the Spanish director Jess Franco (working as Jesús Franco) filmed *Marquis de Sade: Justine*, his own version of Sade's novel, co-starring Klaus Kinski and Romina Power. During the same period, Alejandro Jodorowsky, co-founder of the Panic Movement[5] with the playwright Fernando Arrabal and others, directed *Fando y Lis*, a film based on Jodorowsky's recollections of a play by Arrabal in which two lovers roam a wasteland in search of the mythical city of Tar. When the film was released in Mexico, the work was regarded as so violent, nihilistic, and unnatural that Jodorowsky had to flee the country to escape a lynch mob.

A film shot in Spain in the 1970s—*Tamaño Natural* (1974), by Luis García Berlanga—is one of the most accomplished cinematic portraits of a fetishist. Michel Piccoli plays a dentist who falls in love with a sex doll that becomes his girlfriend, for all practical purposes, since the dentist totally integrates the doll into his daily life. Also in 1974, Don Edmonds directed *Ilsa, She Wolf of the SS*, a Nazi exploitation film loosely based on actual events that occurred in the Buchenwald and Majdanek concentration camps and involved Ilse Koch, the sadistic, lustful wife of these camps' commandant. Another movie with Nazi characters is Tinto Brass's *Los Burdeles de Paprika*, one of this director's most popular films. Bigas Luna gave his sadomasochistic impulses free rein in *Bilbao*, and Buñuel, in his brilliant *That Obscure Object of Desire*, used Sade's *Justine* to elaborate the tenets of his own take on Sade's "misfortunes of virtue" doctrine (the kinder we are to others, the more wicked they are with us, and vice versa). Pier Paolo Pasolini's films in general—and in particular his *Salò, or the 120 Days of Sodom*, nearly two hours of torture and humiliation—are usually also counted among S&M-themed movies.

Pedro Almodóvar was in his glory in the 1980s and early 1990s, thanks in part to two films dealing with sex—*Matador*, whose main characters derive sexual pleasure from killing the objects of their desire, and *Tie Me Up! Tie Me Down!* (1990), in which Antonio Banderas keeps Victoria Abril tied to his bed while a strange, very intense love story plays out between them.

In 1992, the cult director Monika Treut's *Female Misbehavior* was released. Almost four hours long, and consisting of four short documentaries, the film explores the fringes of lesbian behavior and sexuality by focusing on four different women who challenge the status quo, one of whom discusses her sadomasochistic practices from a feminist point of view. Treut took the latter theme up again in *Didn't Do It for Love* (1997), her biopic about Eva Norvind, a Norwegian writer, sex therapist, actress, and dominatrix who lived in Mexico.[6]

David Cronenberg, of course, takes his place as another chronicler of the fetishistic imagination with *Crash*, a film whose characters (James Spader and Holly Hunter, among others) get turned on by the scars and mutilation suffered in car accidents, and by the accidents themselves.

When it comes to contemporary mainstream movies, Isabelle Huppert is my favorite S&M actress (for the

124

classics, Catherine Deneuve is my favorite), since Huppert has appeared in two films that absolutely must be seen, *La Pianiste* and *Ma Mère*, playing women at the mercy of their complicated sexuality (the first is tortured by her passionate sexuality, and the latter is drawn into incest).

And when it comes to movies made for adults, I highly recommend the films of Maria Beatty, whose Bleu Productions (www.bleuproductions.com) gives us exquisitely filmed BDSM relationships between women. Among the actresses who regularly appear in Beatty's films is Midori (www.planetmidori.com), a renowned performer who has written several books on the art of Japanese bondage. There are also some new and interesting filmmakers coming onto the scene, such as Madison Young (www.madisonbound.com), whose debut film, *Bondage Boob Tube*, was named Hottest Kink Film at the 2007 Feminist Porn Awards, and Mistress Basia (www.planetbasia.com), a dominatrix who makes creative, bondage-themed shorts.

Obviously, there are many more movies dealing with themes like submission, role playing, and the cult of pain than these, whose titles I basically came up with off the top of my head. But many women are put off by this genre because, unfortunately, it's still so heavily tilted toward films in which women are dominated and men are the dominators. Oddly enough, things are usually the other way around in the actual S&M scene. Why is that? Let's give it some thought—and then let's get busy!

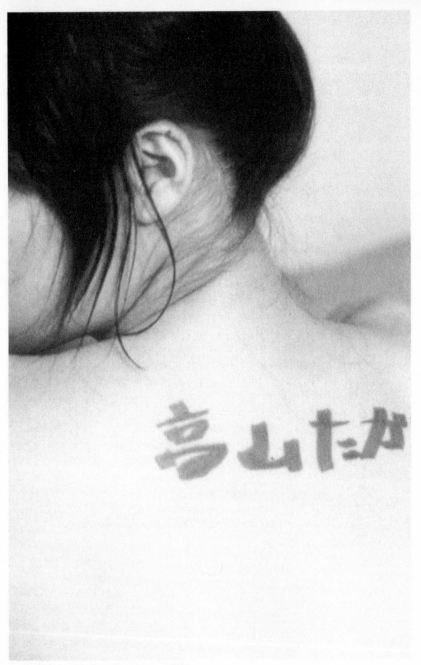

Poster for *Uncle's Paradise* (Japan, 2006)

HENTAI AND OTHER ASIAN FLAVORS

Sex in the Land of the Rising Sun

The Japanese are famous for a sexuality as delicate as it is twisted and morbid. The ancestral culture of the geishas, or pleasure maidens (women whose job it was to provide entertainment of all kinds, including sex, of course), the various types of bondage created to combine submission with pleasure, a highly aesthetic view of fetishism—all these are what make the Japanese true sexual sybarites.

Porn from Japan is popular not only because of its refinement and exoticism but also because of how easily it manages, with a little help from *manga*—and *anime*-style cartoon characters,[7] to breach the barriers erected by self-righteous moralism. Both *manga* and *anime* include a pornographic subgenre, very popular among teenagers (and somewhat older fans), called *hentai* (the word can be translated as both "perversion" and "transformation"). *Hentai* is a term used in connection with extreme and anomalous sexual activities, such as rapes perpetrated by massively well-hung human or fantastic beings, sex with minors, and many other perversions that flesh-and-blood characters could not commit, either for physical reasons or for reasons having to do with the Japanese justice system.

In fact, when it comes to skirting the law, the *hentai* genre is a brilliant example of human ingenuity. Most of the genre's characteristic traits are the products of various legal loopholes. For example, the fact that the characters in many of these films don't have pubic hair is not an indication that they are prepubescent adolescents or children. It's simply a broad-brush solution to a Japanese law, abolished in 1994, against showing pubic hair. Likewise, those imaginary monsters with their famously phallic tentacles are another way

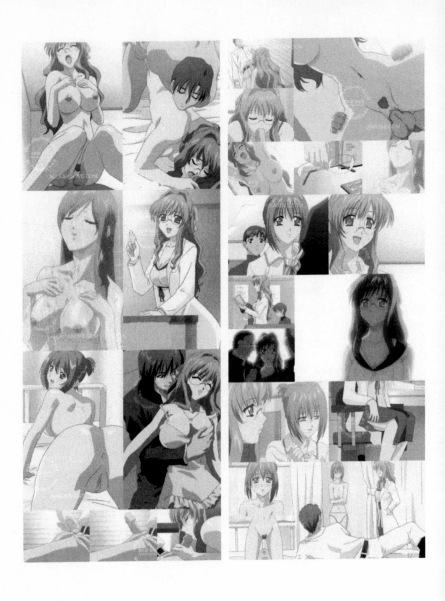

of getting around the law—in this case, a statute against showing male genitals.

The first *manga* artist to depict nude figures was Go Nagai in his *Harenchi Gakuen* series, which was published between 1968 and 1970 but ceased publication because of pressure exerted by parents' associations concerned about possible moral harm to children. From that point on, in parallel with erotic comics in the West (where artists like Guido Crepax and R. Crumb were making their debuts), there were more and more nudes in *manga*, for purely erotic as well as narrative purposes. The freedom to depict nude bodies was hard won in Japan. In a 1976 case, which established a clear cultural precedent, even Oshima Nagisa, director of *In the Realm of the Senses*, was charged with obscenity, and it took six years for his name to be cleared.

The mid-1980s saw the release of the first *hentai* to be sold as an original video animation— *Cream Lemon*, intended for an adult audience.[8] Now the path was clear not just for *hentai* magazines, graphic novels, and films but also for *hentai* video games and all manner of related products. In the 1990s, *hentai* fever struck outside Japan, and works like Hideki Takayama's six-film series *Urotsukidoji: The Legend of the Overfriend*, which pioneered rape-by-tentacle, attained the status of cult movies.

Another type of Japanese erotica, this time with flesh-and-blood characters, is the pink film, a type of characteristically theatrical, humorous softcore pornography most closely related to what we know in the West as sexploitation films. The first pink films were made in the early 1960s, in the restrictive legal environment we've been discussing, and most of these works take pains to elude the censors (for example, by artfully avoiding close-ups of genitals).

According to Jeff Hawkins, executive director of *Hustler*'s Asian Fever, it's interesting that today's trendy Japanese porn, after years of using Gothic Lolitas, refined S&M, golden showers, and all kinds of tools for sexual torture, is now much more like European and American adult films, but with Japanese stars. But the adult film industry in Japan must know what it's doing, since it seems to be making off with some 10 percent of the world market. In spite of censorship and legal complications, the Land of the Rising Sun has become a world-class empire of porn.

 SEX EDUCATION

Any Excuse to Look at Naked Girls

The birth, back in the 1950s, of erotic films for general audiences was certainly not without complications. Public morality (and censorship, in some countries) made producing adult content a complex, risky venture. But every law has its loophole, as they say, and production companies and directors went to great lengths coming up with alibis to get around these problems.

First came nudist films, movies purporting to show both the superiority of the nudist lifestyle, which was then at its peak, and the contentment of the people (almost all of whom happened to be young women with perfect boobs) who had chosen to go through life without a stitch. But the plots of these films quickly wore thin—there's not much of a market for hour-long movies about a voluptuous blonde airing her butt while chasing a beach ball across the sand.

Producers and directors had to dig deeper, and that's when they hit pay dirt. What they came up with was sex education films, movies that are mostly unknown today except as curiosities. These films, purportedly made for strictly hygienic and instructional purposes, demonstrated everything from correct condom use to fungus prevention through proper genital cleansing (as if that would get anybody hot and bothered) to complete sex acts.

Another approach was to demonstrate the terrible consequences of doing something that was clearly forbidden (and if these films are to be believed, it was only the good girls who did such things). Get into a strange man's car, and get yourself raped. Meet some dreamboat in a bar, let him buy you a drink, get yourself raped. Open the door for the meter reader, get yourself raped. Ask some man the time of day, get yourself—guess what—raped. After your prom, get a little tipsy, climb into bed with your classmate, and this will be the one time you won't get yourself raped, but you will get yourself pregnant—also not too shabby, as teen traumas go. In short, there was no excuse too flimsy for staging an erotic scene and showing tits and ass.

Very few of these films achieved any degree of fame, but one of them deserves mention as much for its delectable 1970s aesthetic as for its sound track and the artlessness of its story line. That film is *Schulmädchen-Report: Was Eltern nicht für möglich halten* (literally, *Schoolgirl Report: What Parents Don't Think Is Possible*), the first of a series of sexploitation films by the German director Ernst Hofbauer, which presented the sex lives of twelve teenage girls involved in perpetrating such terrible crimes as rolling around with high school basketball players and opening the door for an alleged doctor who says he's come to offer a vaccination. This film and its sequels were released straight into mainstream movie theaters, and they stayed in the top ten for weeks at a time, earning equal amounts of praise from viewers and indifference from critics. Time heals all things, of course, and time has given these films their due, elevating them to the cult status that should have been theirs to begin with.

Sex education films for adults still exist, but they no longer need excuses of any kind, and they have a very different focus. Instead of teaching you what not to do, a sex education film today is something like a digital Kama Sutra, teaching you how to sharpen your sexual skills so you can give the perfect blow job or perfect the art of anal sex or even undress in a provocative way.

Some of these films are nothing more than compilations of close-ups that demonstrate methods for mastering female ejaculation, marvelous techniques for anal or genital massage to make you see stars, or the best ways to play with your sex toys. Others might feature a porn actress serving as mistress of ceremonies and simply as the master, teaching you all about her best subject—sex.

Nina Hartley, an actress, director, and sex educator, is a regular sex-ed–film machine with her line of instructional videos. At various times in her acting career she has played a guide—to oral sex, orgies, bondage, and threesomes (two guys and a girl, and two girls and a guy) as well as to the topic of her funny and entertaining *Nina Hartley's Guide to Double Penetration*. We should also mention Carol Queen, founder of the prestigious, trailblazing shop Good Vibrations. Queen, along with Shar Rednour and Jackie Strano, is coproducer of the *Bend Over Boyfriend* series, which teaches strap-on use to couples. There is also Betty Dodson, whose films guide women toward better orgasms. And finally we have Tristan Taormino, whose new line of instructional videos for Vivid-Ed got her named Smutty Schoolteacher of the Year at the 2008 Feminist Porn Awards.

DOCUMENTARIES

Up Close and Intimate

The world of adult films also includes documentaries—movies that portray intimacy between real people, showing who these people are as well as their opinions and their experiences of love and sex. People who truly don't like porn may still like sexually explicit documentaries, since these films don't rely on histrionics or exaggeration. Films dealing with minority issues and viewpoints fall into this genre, and so do works focused on key moments in the history of pornographic film. The purpose of some documentaries is to arouse the viewer. Others portray sex in a natural and authentic way, and still others examine human sexual behavior without intruding on the action.

Annie Sprinkle's *Herstory of Porn*

The legendary Annie Sprinkle—porn actress and performance artist, feminist, postpornographic philosopher, and more—journeys back in time to show us the best (and the worst) sex scenes she has acted in through more than two decades, and more than 150 movies, in the world of adult films. This masterful documentary, based on one of Sprinkle's monologues, is an interesting eyewitness account of that mythical era known as the sexual revolution.

Thinking XXX

From Savanna Samson to Nina Hartley, from straights to gays, and from veterans to newcomers, *Thinking XXX* takes an unvarnished look at some legendary figures of North American porn. These men and women were interviewed on camera in New York and Los Angeles while they were posing for *XXX: 30 Porn-Star Portraits*, a unique book by the photographer Timothy Greenfield-Sanders that reflects on the world

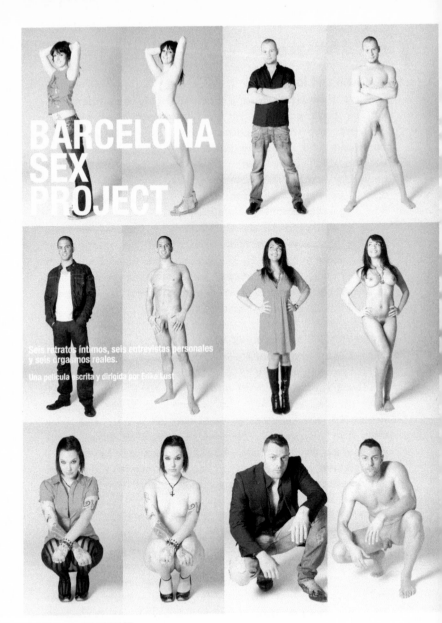

BARCELONA SEX PROJECT
Six intimate portraits, six personal interviews, and six real orgasms
A film written and directed by Erika Lust

of porn and includes essays by J. T. Leroy, John Malkovich, John Waters, Salman Rushdie, and Lou Reed, among others. In this documentary we see the stars discussing exhibitionism, public and private sex, money, and today's porn business. Interviewed in their homes, at their offices, or at the gym, in the company of their husbands and wives, their friends and lovers, they share their worries, their thoughts about the sex industry, and their hopes and dreams.

The Beautiful Agony of Orgasm

The Internet is home to a proliferation of erotic and sexually explicit websites that double as Internet 2.0 social networking sites, where users create the content. For that reason, the Internet has also become an excellent platform for a new type of documentary, in which viewers can also become performers. In the world of these do-it-yourself (DIY) documentaries, the most remarkable phenomenon is a venture based in Melbourne, Australia, which originally created the website I Shot Myself (www.ishotmyself.com), followed by Beautiful Agony (www.beautifulagony.com), and, finally, I Feel Myself (www.ifeelmyself.com). All three sites subscribe to the DIY philosophy, and all three feature plenty of bold women (plus a few men) who take pleasure in their sexuality and their bodies. They are students, workers, and travelers, widowed and married, of diverse ethnicities, ages, sexualities, bodies, and mind-sets. They are uniquely themselves, and they want to free their sexuality by displaying it in public, in a natural way.

Comstock Films

This production company, founded by the husband-and-wife team of Tony and Peggy Comstock, offers an authentic look at sex with a partner in a series of explicit documentaries showing real people having real sex on camera. With these depictions of actual sex, in which narrative and cinematic aims play no part, Comstock has produced a documentary genre that falls halfway between art and pornography. But these works are not strictly about sex. "Flesh without context is of no more interest to me than sex without love," says Tony Comstock. "In my films, context is provided by an intimate conversation with each couple that is, in some ways, more revealing than the sex."[9] The productions from Comstock Films offer a new vision of eroticism as well as an exploration and celebration of human sexual experience.

Tristan Taormino's *Chemistry*

Documentary or reality porn? Imagine an unfiltered, intimate, personal look at sex among seven people who know themselves and know what they like. For a new perspective on adult documentaries, the postfeminist and postporn activist Tristan Taormino offers the use of her camera. And for her *Chemistry* series, she left groups of women and men locked in a house for two days, free to do as they pleased with whomever they chose. In addition to sex, the films feature intimate confessions made to the camera by each of the participants in this documentary experiment.

Morty Diamond's *Trans Entities*

Trans Entities: The Nasty Love of Papí and Wil is a documentary about a transgender couple, and it's one of the few that not only includes sex but also manages to be both provocative and moving. In this film directed by Morty Diamond, Papí and Wil seem completely natural and free of hang-ups as they show us their reality and their ordinariness as a couple. According to Diamond, "They are a perverted,

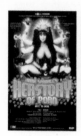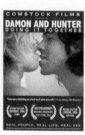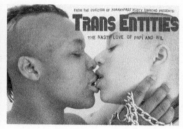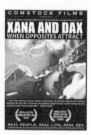

loving, polyamorous couple who identify as Trans Entities, a word they have coined to describe their gender identity. Armed with my video camera, I set out to capture this couple in a multifaceted way, from revealingly personal interviews to fun nights out on the town. The three sex scenes in the movie, including one with a third partner, were shot completely undirected, allowing the viewer an engagingly raw look into their uninhibited exploration of role playing, BDSM, and lots of hot sex."[10]

Barcelona Sex Project

My latest film, *Barcelona Sex Project* (www.barcelona sexproject.com), falls squarely into the genre we've been discussing—the erotic documentary. In *Barcelona Sex Project*, I offer an intimate, unmediated look at three men and three women—their lives, and even their actual orgasms—so the viewer can really get to know them. They share their thoughts, passions, and reflections in personal interviews, and each of them carries a camera around to present his or her daily life in a natural way. Finally, in individual masturbation scenes, they all invite us to take a peek at their most private, intimate pleasure. The people who appear in this movie are David Galant, Joni Lapaz, Joel Acosta, Dunia Montenegro, Irina Vega, and Silvia Rubí. Thanks to La Maleta Roja; to Jailhousefuck for an incredible bed; and to Late Chocolate for the Late Late.[11]

ALT-PORN

Sneakers, Dreads, and Piercings:
Erotic Potential Unleashed

Mention the words *porn actress,* and most people won't have any trouble coming up with the image of a woman, size 8, with enormous breasts, full lips, luxuriant hair, and a perfect bikini wax. And that's the way it was all through the 1980s and much of the 1990s, until the advent of alternative porn, or alt-porn, a type of adult entertainment directed at the alt subculture. Alt-porn arose in response to market demand for a new and more modern erotica that would appeal to the new urban tribes.

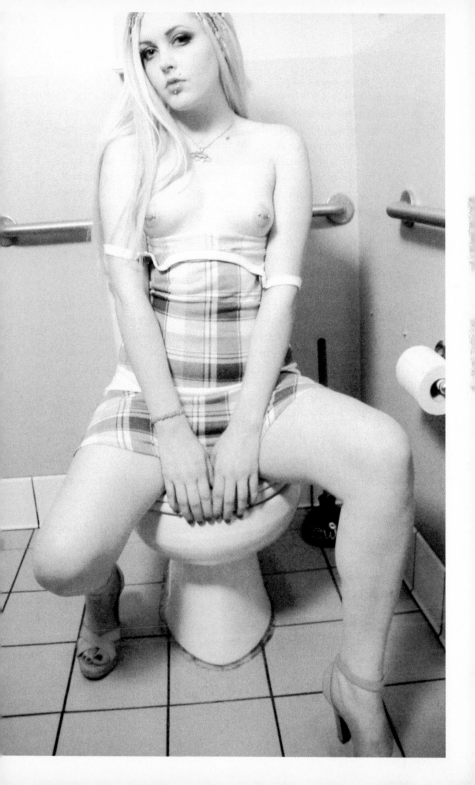

The best way to tell if you're watching an alt-porn movie or looking at alt-porn photographs is to count the number and kinds of tattoos on the women. If a woman has a *Playboy* bunny tattooed on her groin, you're looking at mainstream porn; likewise if she has a rose on her butt. But if she has a pair of 1950s-style swallows on her shoulders, a tribal tattoo on her tailbone, a couple of Maori bracelet tattoos, three pinup tattoos on her arms and legs, and a variety of piercings to top it all off, there's no question that this is an alt production. Her hair is also likely to be styled in makeshift dreadlocks or dyed some impossible color, or she'll have a Mohawk or even a shaved head.

Little by little, the boldest and trendiest adult boutiques have been making room for alt-porn, but most of these videos and photographs are sold on the Internet, even though the genre got its start in a print-based publication, *Blue Blood* magazine. Most of the models in alt-porn photography are not professionals but nameless girls who at some point just felt like having some erotic photos taken, or maybe they took the photos themselves. Regardless, the outcome is seldom a career in porn, a fact that accounts for another of alt-porn's characteristics—unretouched photos. Alt-porn has plump girls with Coke-bottle glasses and huge breasts, and it has girls with pink dreads who are flat as a board. In the alt world, both looks are considered valid and attractive.

For a sample of these looks, check out Suicide Girls (www.suicidegirls.com), possibly the most famous alt-porn website. By the site's own account, Suicide Girls is where you'll find the world's most beautiful alternative pinups. Suicide Girls operates on a members-only basis. Its intentions are not so much pornographic as artistic and erotic (for example, there are very few spread shots, and there are no images of penetration, although lesbians are represented), and it offers everything from Gothic Lolitas in thongs to blue-haired Asians and actual punk rockers with three nipple rings.

Given how successful and lucrative this business can be, the growth in online alternative photo galleries has been exponential, creating conditions ripe for the appearance of sites like Deviant Nation (www.deviantnation.com), Barely Evil (www.barelyevil.com), and God's Girls (www.gods girls.com, from the creators of Suicide Girls but with an elegant, classy touch).

The websites just discussed are basically devoted to still photography, but on the video-based Burning Angel (www.burningangel.com) girls upload short homemade clips of themselves masturbating alone, or clips of themselves with other girls as well as with guys. Audience response has been so favorable that Burning Angel was encouraged to establish a production company that goes by the same name, and its first film was the gonzo feature *Cum On My Tattoo*, starring its director, Joanna Angel. Burning Angel is now in the process of designing a line of alt sex toys—and, really, what better accessory for a punk rock girl than a leopard-print vibrator to go with her skateboard?

One of the few directors to have made a name for himself in alt-porn is Eon McKai, an American enamored of punk rock. When he was only twenty-five, McKai directed his first film, *Art School Sluts*, in which performers with a totally indie look have sex in classrooms. Short pleated skirts, teddy bears, safety pins, Converse sneakers, and bitten-down nails with chipped polish have entered the alternative erotic imagination because of this film, which also features terrific art direction as well as a screenplay that pushes alt-porn beyond pure and simple gonzo.

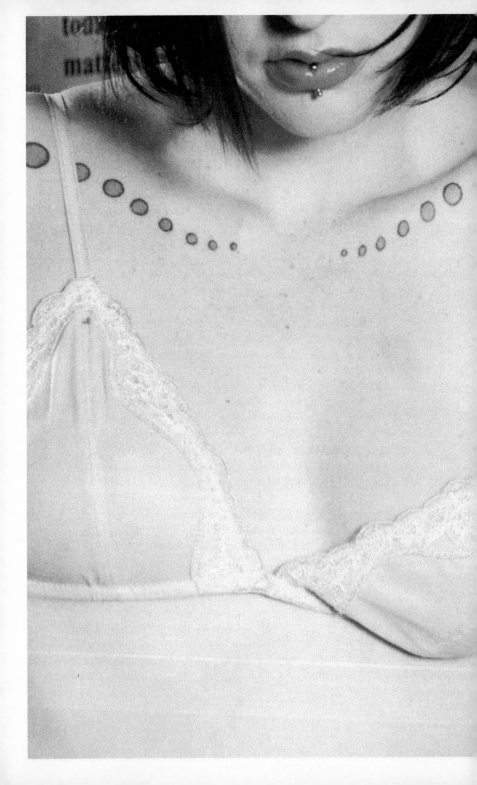

McKai later signed with the Vivid-Alt division of Vivid Entertainment (www.vividalt.com), a production company that has placed its bet on alt-porn as the wave of a different, better future. Other directors active in the company are Dave Naz (who made *Skater Girl Fever* and is a true fan of girls on wheels); the artist Vena Virago; the self-described paranoid and compulsive Dana DeArmond, who also writes and acts in her films; and the photographer Winky Tiki, who flawlessly re-creates the 1950s pinup aesthetic.

Anyone who doubts how good things are right now for this kind of adult entertainment only has to take a look at how many alt-porn festivals are popping up all over the world. Whether it's the section dedicated to alt-porn at the Los Angeles Erotica Film Fest, or PornfilmfestivalBerlin's Cum2Cut competition, which invites contestants to use their own bodies to demonstrate new ways of presenting erotic material, or the Amsterdam Alternative Erotica Film Festival, there are more and more signs that porn has come a long way from silicone-enhanced, Brazilian-waxed blondes and is starting to notice erotic piercing, tattoos, and dirty sneakers.

 HARDCORE ART FILMS

From Bergman to Mitchell

When film became a means of mass communication, back in the 1930s, conservative forces in Western societies quickly mobilized to regulate it, especially in matters that involved sex. They created bodies for censorship and control, to dictate what filmmakers could and could not show on the screen. To get around the censors, many filmmakers resorted to metaphor. In one shot, for example, a couple would be kissing and

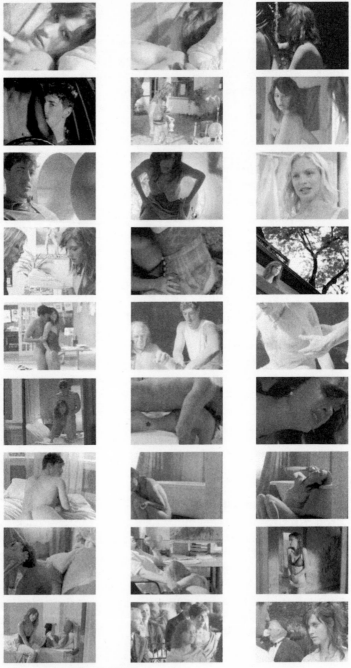

Screen shots from *Lie with Me* (2005)

on the verge of making love, and in the next shot a speeding train would enter a tunnel—an obvious allusion to penetration. All of this is shown beautifully in the 1995 documentary *The Celluloid Closet*, based on the book by Vito Russo and written and directed by Rob Epstein and Jeffrey Friedman. The film does a superb job of describing the repressive atmosphere that enveloped the big Hollywood studios, and it explains the narrative and visual codes that screenwriters and producers invented to indicate that certain characters were gay.

While the censors were tightening the screws in the United States, with the Motion Picture Association of America (MPAA) serving as standard bearer for ultraconservative moralism, sex was beginning to be portrayed more freely and more naturally in European and Asian independent films. Movies like Michelangelo Antonioni's *Blow Up*, Luis Buñuel's *Belle de Jour*, Ingmar Bergman's *Summer with Monika*, Oshima Nagisa's *In the Realm of the Senses*, and Bernardo Bertolucci's *Last Tango in Paris* are good examples of the reaction against prudish Hollywood productions.

One point worth noting is that because pornography is defined as entertainment whose ultimate goal is the viewer's sexual arousal, the films just mentioned are different in principle from porn. They don't shrink from graphic representations of sex, but they also don't use sex simply to arouse the spectator. They use it to tell a story. In keeping with this trend, the 1990s saw the emergence of a new film genre devoted to portraying sex openly, but without the viewer's arousal as its ultimate goal. Directors like Michael Winterbottom, Catherine Breillat, Lars von Trier, Todd Solondz, Bernardo Bertolucci, Gaspar Noé, Patrice Chéreau, and John Cameron Mitchell have defied the pretty prism of softcore Hollywood sex. Linda Williams, writing about this kind of movie in her book *Screening Sex*, says, "The films of hard-core art may be aggressive, violent, humiliating, desperate, alienating, tender, loving, playful, joyous and, of course, boring, but they are art films that . . . embrace explicit sexual content."[12]

HERE ARE SOME DIRECTORS (AS USUAL, THERE ARE ONLY A FEW WOMEN) WHOSE MOVIES DON'T KEEP SEX UNDER WRAPS

Ingmar Bergman	Lars von Trier
Vilgot Sjöman	Todd Solondz
Oshima Nagisa	Gaspar Noé
Luis Buñuel	Clement Virgo
Michelangelo Antonioni	Steven Shainberg
Bernardo Bertolucci	Kimberly Peirce
Patrice Chéreau	Vincent Gallo
Catherine Breillat	Julio Medem
Virginie Despentes	Bigas Luna
Jane Campion	David Lynch
Roman Polanski	Ziad Doueiri
Jean-Jacques Annaud	Michael Winterbottom
Michael Haneke	John Cameron Mitchell

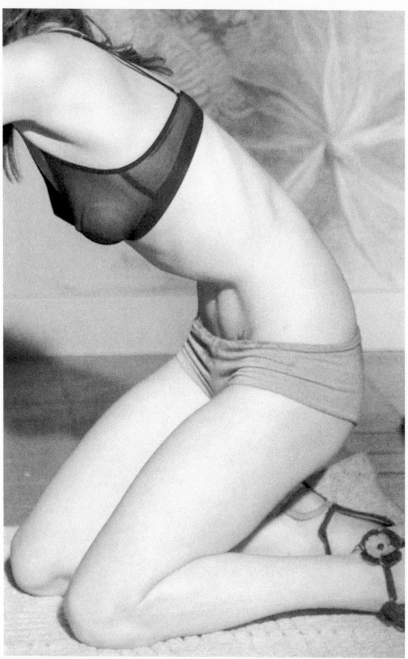

Lie with Me (2005)

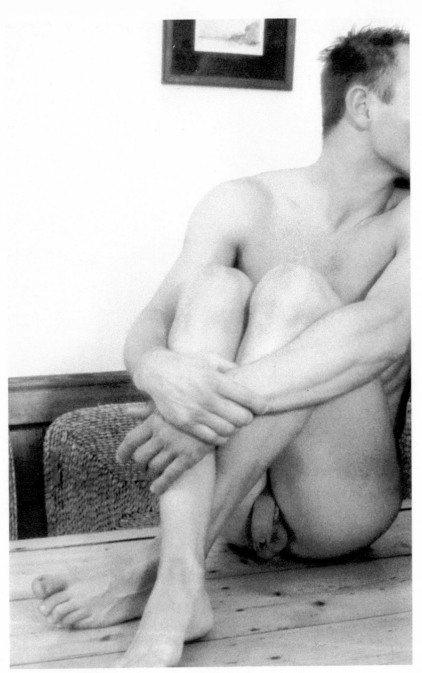

Anna's Mates (2002)

NEW WAVE PORN

Art, Film, Porn, or All Three?

Let's take a look at the phenomenon of independent artists and producers who are using traditional pornography as a vehicle for critical reflection, and who are also looking for new and creative ways of including sexual content in their films.

According to Beatriz Preciado, "Toward the end of the 1990s, a number of French porn actors and actresses began to produce their own films and develop critical perspectives on their profession, a phenomenon that gave rise to an unprecedented way of representing sexuality. To borrow a phrase from André Bazin, we might call it New Wave porn."[13] These artists elude strict classification as either pornographers or filmmakers. Taking their inspiration from trashy novels as well as from Charles Baudelaire, Charles Bukowski, and Lydia Lunch, from horror films and the punk and goth subcultures, and from sex-positive strains of American feminism and Annie Sprinkle's critiques of

149

traditional porn, they've thrown in their lot with a new politics of the gaze.[14]

But this development hasn't been limited to porn industry insiders. Many young people from all over the world, and from backgrounds in a variety of disciplines outside adult entertainment, have also been turning a modern critical eye on the business. Among filmmakers, this new movement includes some young women, who finally don't have to feel put off or degraded by porn. Instead, they're joining the New Wave movement with enthusiasm and bringing a new feminine, and feminist, outlook.

I count myself among them, and I like to think that we are the future of this minirevolution whose job it is to help transform adult entertainment, not only by bringing it up to date but also by turning it into something that women as well as men can accept and enjoy. This section presents a few of these artists. It's not an exhaustive list, but it does introduce you to a selection of those who have done the most outstanding work over the past few years.

Maria Beatty
(www.bleuproductions.com)
Born in Venezuela, brought up in New York, and now living in Paris, this sophisticated woman has directed and occasionally acted in more than twenty-five short films with lesbian/S&M themes. Every film directed by Beatty has meticulous cinematography and an elaborate cinematic idiom.

Bruce LaBruce
(www.brucelabruce.com)
Bruce LaBruce is a controversial Canadian writer, photographer, director, and gay underground porn actor. His films include *The Raspberry Reich*, *Skin Flick*, *Hustler White*, *Super 8? No Skin Off My Ass*, and *Boy, Girl*.

Anna Span
(www.annaspansdiary.com)

This director has established herself as one of the most prolific creators of the new adult films in Britain. She has directed *Anna's Mates, Uniform Behaviour, Toy with Me*, and *Good Service*, among other films.

Innocent Pictures
(www.innocentpictures.com)

This adult film production company was originally a subsidiary of the famed Danish director Lars Von Trier's company, and today it has several titles on the market, among them *All About Anna, Constance*, and *Pink Prison*. One of the company's founders, Nicholas Barbano, is also the author of *The Puzzy Power Manifesto*, an compelling statement on the new adult films.

Petra Joy
(www.petrajoy.com)

Petra was born in Germany and now lives in Brighton (UK). Her production company Strawberry Seductress has released three female-oriented titles: *Sexual Sushi, Female Fantasies*, and *Feeling It!*

Jennifer Lyon Bell
(www.blueartichokefilms.com)

This American director, now living in Amsterdam, is the founder of Blue Artichoke Films. She brings a refreshing intellectual vision to the world of adult films. Her short film *Headshot* is a good example of that vision, and her second film, *Matinée*, was released in 2009.

Ovidie
(www.pornomanifesto.com)

Ovidie, a French porn actress, producer, and director, was born in 1980. While she was still a philosophy student, she wrote two books about her involvement in the world of porn, *Porno Manifesto* and *In Sex We Trust: Backstage*. Her credits as a director and producer include, most notably, *Orgie en Noir* and *Lilith*.

HPG
(www.hpgnet.com)
Hervé Pierre Gustav is a porn actor, producer, and director. He is one of the most controversial figures in the French adult film industry, since his work contains so much dark humor and self-abasement. In 2005, his film *On ne devrait pas exister* was accepted for screening at the Cannes Film Festival.

Roy Stuart
(www.roystuart.net)
This American photographer, now settled in Paris, has published several books with Taschen. His photographs and films are characterized by a delicate blend of glamour and pornography that highlights female beauty and a BDSM aesthetic.

Mia Engberg
(www.miaengberg.com)
This Swedish director is laying claim to a new, feminist porn. She has directed several short films, most notably *Selma & Sofie*, and was recently awarded a grant from the Swedish government to produce a feminist pornographic movie called *Dirty Diaries*.

Sofilles Productions
(www.secondsexe.com)
French film producer Sophie Bramly has commissioned several female directors to direct a series of short movies that have been released under the name X-FEMMES. Among the directors are Caroline Loeb,

Lola Doillon, Helena Noguerra, Zoé Cassavetes, Tonie Marshall, and Ann Mouglalis.

Estelle Joseph

Estelle Joseph, founder of Stella Films, is the director of the *City of Flesh* series, films that have been equally successful with mainstream and festival audiences, partly because of the performers' ethnic diversity.

Venus Hottentot
(www.venushottentot.com)

Venus Hottentot is another director who stands out for her ethnically diverse approach. *AfroDite Superstar*, Hottentot's first film, was released through the Femme Chocolat division of Femme Productions, the company run by Candida Royalle, a trailblazer in adult films for women.

Eva Midgley
(www.quietstormfilms.com)

Eva Midgley, director of the award-winning shorts *Honey and Bunny* and the visually beautiful *Footsie*, collaborates with Coco de Mer, the English adult boutique founded by Sam Roddick, daughter of the late Anita Roddick, who herself founded the Body Shop chain. You can see chapters 1 and 2 of *Honey and Bunny* free of charge on YouTube (www.youtube .com) by entering the term *honey and bunny* along with the term *coco-de-mer* in YouTube's search box. More samples of Midgley's work are available for free viewing on the Quiet Storm Films website.

Julia Ostertag
(www.julia-ostertag.de)

This Berlin-based German director has enjoyed great success at alternative film festivals with a short, *Sexjunkie*, and with *Gender X*, a documentary that examines the line between gender and identity.

Émilie Jouvet
(www.myspace.com/hysterieprod;
www.myspace.com/onenightstandmovie
Émilie Jouvet is one of the founders of Hystérie
Prod. Her film *Pour Une Nuit/One-Night Stand* is an ode
to the lesbotrans, boi, and transfag scene in Paris.

New Wave Porn also includes directors like Audacia
Ray and Shine Louise Houston, mentioned earlier in
this chapter and discussed elsewhere in this book
(see chapter 9). In addition, I think the directors
brought together by Eon McKai at Vivid-Alt belong
to the New Wave as well.

Obviously, every day there are more people
joining the New Wave Porn movement. This book
discusses only those artists who have established
themselves in one way or another. If you're interested
in exploring and discovering new talent, check out
the indie, queer, alt, feminist, and amateur porn
festivals that are starting up all over.

 DIY

Sex, Webcams, and Videotape

The British punk rock movement was as much about
fashion as about music and art, and it urged people
of that era to break away from business as usual and
do things themselves by creating their own clothes,
their own songs, and their own role models. Some
thirty years later, all that remains of the movement
in terms of fashion are biker-style wristbands and
studded belts. But when it comes to porn, punk's
message is livelier than ever, especially since the
advent of the Internet.

And when it comes to amateur porn, the do-
it-yourself subgenre, as its name implies, is the

kind you can make on your own, with your video camera and a little help from your partner, your vibrator, or your best friend. Right now, in the middle of the Web 2.0 revolution, you can make love, masturbate, or do a striptease and then, with just a few clicks, and without ever leaving your room, put your images of these activities in front of millions of people. That's why the World Wide Web is usually the distribution point for this subgenre of porn. For a film to be considered truly amateur, the only requirement is that the people who appear in it must not have been paid, or that they don't normally do this kind of thing or do it for a living. So does this mean that gonzo is also a genre of amateur porn? The answer is no. Even though the girls are beginners, and would be classified as amateurs for that reason, the companies behind gonzo productions are obviously professional.

Now that we've cleared that up, let's move on with a little of amateur porn's history. Amateur porn for mass consumption (recall that the first pornographic films were made to order for upper-middle-class and aristocratic men, which makes those films *almost* DIY projects) got its start in magazines published for readers who were looking for sex partners or involved in swinging. For a prospective swinger to have any interest in a person or a couple, the "merchandise" had to be displayed attractively, a necessity that eventually led these magazines to become another source of material for consumers of porn, since the "girl next door" appeal of ordinary women took these magazines beyond the exclusive circle of actual swingers and into the realm of jack-off material. And, really, isn't there a certain sick fascination about watching two people fuck when they look less like Pamela Anderson and Nacho Vidal and more like you and your partner?

Entrepreneurs in this area are not idiots, and they caught on right away. Focusing specifically on adult newsstands and bookstores, they began satisfying the demand for homemade videos and, later, homemade DVDs that were more or less appealing, with better or worse lighting and more or less decent screenplays, or no screenplays at all. But the newsstand- and bookstore-based amateurs' days were numbered. As use of the Internet continued to spread, every home soon had a computer and a modem (even if it was only a 52K contraption that made infernal noises getting connected and cut out every time the phone rang), and this meant that any old computer could now be turned into a small independent production company. And so began the golden age of homemade porn. With the development of items like webcams as well as web-based technologies like streaming video, which allows files to be viewed without having to be downloaded, everything became easier and easier for users.

Websites like www.xtube.com, www.youporn.com, www.yuvutu.com, www.pornotube.com, and any number of other sites with names that combine part of the term *YouTube* (the name of the mother of all streaming sites) with some sort of term related to sex, are places where you can make yourself a star in a matter of seconds—and you'll only be a star for a few seconds, too, since fleeting fame is part and parcel of amateur porn. The consumers of homemade porn are not looking for a star, or for a particular face or cock, or for a recognizable pair of boobs. They're looking for an unrehearsed cock, an anonymous boob, or just ordinary sex between ordinary people, and those who provide it are usually people who feel like acting on the exhibitionism that all of us share, to some extent.

You can also make a movie, or pose for some photos with your partner, for no other reason beyond watching your film or looking at your photos together later on so you can have a record of your erotic moments. A production of your own—maybe one that encourages you to try that position in the video a second or third time, or one that shows you both something about how you make love—can be truly exciting if you can manage to stop focusing on the weight you have to lose (or gain) and treat yourself with more acceptance and respect. After all, what could be more erotic than pleasing yourself?

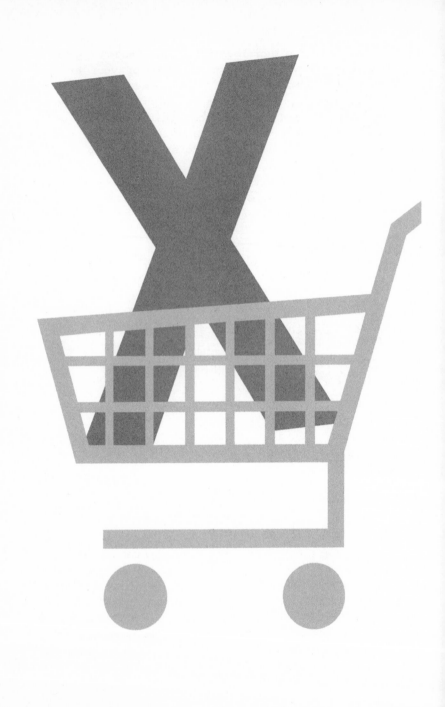

CHAPTER 8
SEXY SHOPPING

We women are coming into our own as a thriving market for sexually oriented products and services. We're revolutionizing the adult entertainment industry, and it seems the industry has realized that we're here, that we have money, that we're sexually liberated, and that we want to have fun and enjoy ourselves—not just as consumers, either. Every day, more and more women entrepreneurs are starting their own businesses. Who knows more than women about what other women like?

DOWN WITH ADULT BOOKSTORES, UP WITH ADULT BOUTIQUES

Why don't I like adult bookstores? Because their storefronts are scary-looking, and the stores are dark inside, with a sinister atmosphere and 128-channel viewing booths that give off a stench of crusted semen mixed with cheap air freshener. You have to walk past fat old bald guys who give you dirty looks, and you can forget about asking the clerks a question—they're usually men you're better off not talking to at all. As for the merchandise, it's next to impossible to find anything you might want. Movies and magazines account for 90 percent of what's on sale, and don't even think about finding anything just for women. The sex toys are still only a sideline, and the few that exist are designed and

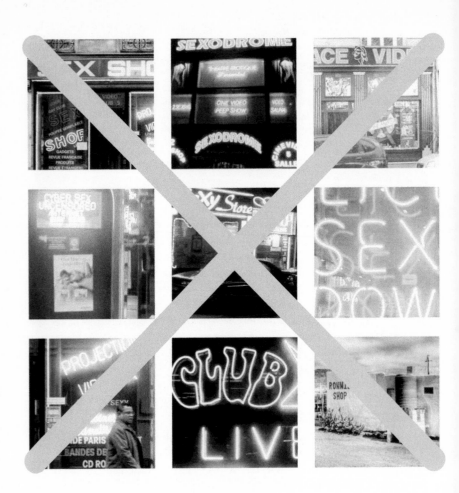

packaged in a way that recalls the worst of the 1980s. Even if you should happen to get lucky and find something to wear, chances are it will be a cheap latex uniform (for a nurse, a policewoman, or a waitress), or maybe you'll come across a pair of edible panties. These adult bookstores are owned by men. They're for male customers, with merchandise meant to satisfy men's desires.

THE NEW ADULT BOUTIQUES
Is there any alternative for women? There certainly is. We have our own places now, on the streets of our cities and on the Internet. And the first thing we've done is change the way we talk about them. These aren't adult bookstores. They're adult boutiques, with attractive storefronts and pretty, well-informed girls behind the counter. They're stylish on the inside, and they sell clothing, candles, and incense. They have fitting rooms, too, where you can try on sensual erotic lingerie, and they sell masks, whips, beautifully designed sex toys, cosmetics with aphrodisiac properties, oils, books, music, movies, jewelry . . . let's see how long it takes the sex and eroticism industry to wise up! We have the potential to be a very important customer base. The new adult boutiques aren't just for women, of course—they have male customers, too—but women are drawn to their ethic and their aesthetic.

These boutiques are usually much more than businesses. Some are also centers for education, reflection, and debate. Many sponsor lectures, talks, classes, seminars, and workshops. One boutique in Toronto, Good for Her (www.goodforher.com), even sponsors the highly regarded Feminist Porn Awards.

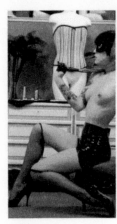

La Juguetería
www.lajugueteria.com
Travesía de San Mateo, 12
Madrid

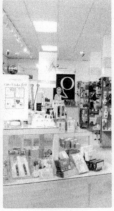

Good Vibrations
www.goodvibes.com
603 Valencia Street
San Francisco,
California 94110

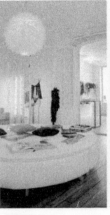

Yoba
www.yobaparis.com
1 Rue du Marché St. Honoré
Paris, France

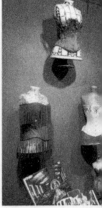

Coco de Mer
www.coco-de-mer.com
23 Monmouth Street
Covent Garden, London W
England

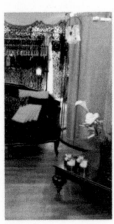

Lust
www.lust.dk
Mikkel Bryggersgade 3A
Copenhagen, Denmark

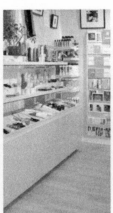

Good for Her
www.goodforher.com
175 Harbord Street
Toronto, Canada

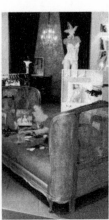

Le Boudoir
www.leboudoir.net
Canuda 21
Barcelona, Spain

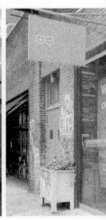

Babeland
www.babeland.com
707 East Pike Street
Seattle, Washington 9812

THE INTERNET: SEXY SHOPPING MADE EASY AND ANONYMOUS

The Internet is one of the adult entertainment industry's best friends. It certainly has increased sales. The ability to use a credit card to buy sexually oriented products from the comfort and anonymity of home has given many people the courage to experiment with items they might not have bought if they had walked into a bricks-and-mortar store.

Walk-in adult boutiques for women have sprouted up in major cities all over the world, and the growth in online boutiques has been even greater. Online boutiques offer products carefully chosen with women in mind—vibrators and toys of all kinds, dildos, books, items for bondage and S&M, lubricants, massage oils, and of course movies. Many of the online boutiques also specialize in films and videos. They carry a good selection of movies that women like, and they offer them with detailed synopses and recommendations from informed reviewers.

WATCHING ADULT FILMS ONLINE: HOW AND WHERE?

Broadband Internet connections and streaming (a technology for watching or listening to media files right on a website) have made it possible to watch videos on your computer without having to download a file or buy a physical copy of a film.

Most streaming film sites use the Pay-Per-View (PPV) system. With PPV, subscribers pay for the individual items they want to see, such as sporting events, recently released movies, major concerts, and, as we've been discussing, X-rated scenes or movies. PPV is also used by cable and satellite TV, another place to find multiple channels of adult entertainment, although most, as always, are focused on men.

agentprovocateur.com
amantis.net
amorspilar.se
annsummers.co.uk
asprix.com
a-womans-touch.com
babeland.com
bedroompleasures.co.uk
blacklabeladultshop.com
blamblam.com
bonkum.com
calexotics.com
camaderosas.com
coco-de-mer.co.uk
comeasyouare.com
cupido.no
desig.org
divine-interventions.com
early2bed.com
eltocador.com
emotionalbliss.com
erotikazamora.com
eternalspirits.com
factormujer.com
femmefatal.de
gash.co.uk
glamorousamorous.com
goodforher.com
goodvibes.com
grandopening.com
hysteriashop.com
indulgeparty.com
jimmyjane.com

kikidm.com
ladybliss.com
lajugueteria.com
lamaletaroja.com
lamusardine.com
latechocolate.com
leboudoir.net
leroidelacapote.com
losplaceresdelola.com
lossecretosdemiflor.co
lovehoney.co.uk
lovestore.nu
lust.dk
lustjakt.se
mailfemale.com
manomarabotti.com
melroseurbanfemale.com
mikoretail.com
moilafemme.com
morbia.com
mosexstore.com
mutine.fr
myla.com
nudgenudge.com
passion8.co.uk
pinkpomelo.es
pkwholesalers.com
pussydeluxe.de
scarletssecrets.co.uk
secondsexe.com
selfservetoys.com
sexapilas.com
sextoys.co.uk
sexybank.es
shesaidboutique.com
shespot.nl
sh-womenstore.com
softparis.com
stockroom.com
suicidegirls.com/shop
thepleasurechest.com
tiendadurex.com
topersex.com
venusenvy.ca
vibrator.com
whysleep.co.uk
xandria.com
yobaparis.com

Here are a few outstanding online video membership sites.

Hot Movies for Her

At Hot Movies for Her (www.hotmoviesforher.com), you pay by the minute and can choose from an extensive and diverse video library in a large number of categories (for example, Feminist Porn Award winners).

I Feel Myself

I heartily recommend www.ifeelmyself.com. Though not exactly X-rated, it has thousands of fresh, natural, modern masturbation scenes showing women feeling sexual pleasure and having real orgasms. Membership plans start at less than $30 per month.

Retro and Vintage Porn

At www.vintagepayperview.com, affiliated with the streaming video giant AEBN (Adult Entertainment Broadcast Network), you can browse porn classics—great films of the 1970s and early 1980s, the golden age of porn. Personally, I really like these older films from a time when adult movies still had a certain innocence as well as plots that were much more imaginative than they are today.

Seconde Sex's Médiathèque

Seconde Sex may be the most innovative online adult boutique in France, and possibly in all of Europe. At www.secondesex.com you'll find a good selection of movies, including some of Seconde Sex's own productions.

Good Vibrations' Video on Demand (VOD)

Good Vibrations, one of the first U.S. adult boutiques for women, has also launched an online VOD service at www.goodvibes.com.

Babeland VOD

Babeland, with its original store in Seattle and three branches in New York (Brooklyn, the Lower East Side, and SoHo), is another trailblazer in the sale of movies and other products designed for women, both in the Babeland stores and on the Internet (www.babeland.com).

Lust Cinema

These are my own movies, which include Five Hot Stories for Her, Barcelona Sex Project, Handcuffs and Life, and Love & Lust. All are available for stream or download at www.lustcinema.com.

TIP

To keep up with the latest innovations and wildest oddities in adult entertainment, visit www.fleshbot .com once in a while. Over the past few years, this site has become the online bible for all things erotic and pornographic.

For Free

One of men's specialties—and men have a years-long head start on us—is watching and bootlegging Internet porn. Just as you can download movies through peer-to-peer (P2P) file-sharing software like BitTorrent and eMule, you can go to sites like www.xvideos.com, www.redtube.com, www.pornhub.com, www.xtube.com, and www.megarotic.com to watch porn online without downloading it onto your computer. But most of the offerings are miniclips or scenes from gonzo porn, and the production values usually leave quite a bit to be desired. You won't be breaking any laws if you visit these sites, but you won't find entire movies, either, and there won't be much for you to choose from, or at least not much of anything you might actually want to see. What you'll find instead is a potpourri of rough, hardcore sex.

THE "TUPPERSEX" PARTY: A HOME-BASED ADULT BOUTIQUE

It all started with Tupperware, the food-storage containers, unique in their day, that were famous not only for being the first product of their kind but also for being marketed and promoted at parties held in women's homes.

This home-based approach to sales soon spread

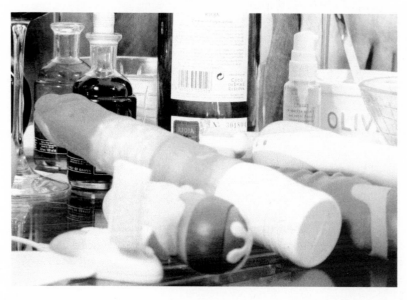

to other types of products that until recently
were the exclusive province of women (cosmetics,
kitchenware, and the like). But women have evolved,
and so have home parties. These days they're used
to sell sex toys, and women gather to share and
compare their experiences with various products.

Home parties are held regularly in England
and the United States. One American company
specializing in home parties is Passion Parties
(www.passionparties.com), with a network of sales
reps working across the country. The advantage of
a "Tuppersex" party is that women don't have to
deal with the discomfort that some might feel about
visiting a commercial establishment.

FILM FESTIVALS: ANOTHER WAY TO WATCH

The democratization of audiovisual production has
had effects that can be seen in the adult film
industry. The world of pornographic movies now
encompasses the efforts of many young filmmakers from
all over the world, who bring a fresh perspective
unspoiled by the clichés of tradtional porn.

Many of these filmmakers are shooting commercial
adult movies, but quite a few are simply experimenting
and making films with the freedom afforded by not
having to market their work. One result has been the
emergence of hundreds of new festivals to welcome
this new phenomenon, known as art-house porn or, as
some prefer, indie or New Wave porn.

Major Adult Film Festivals
Venus
Berlin
www.venus-berlin.com
This is another major European festival, held every
year in October. With more than thirty-five countries

represented, and with four hundred exhibitors gathered at the 300,000-square-foot festival site, this event is a must.

AVN Awards and Expo
Las Vegas
www.avnawards.com
The AVN Awards, sponsored by the trade magazine *Adult Video News*, are the adult film industry's biggest event—the Oscars of X-rated films, with the world's most important stars on the red carpet, and the distinctive glamour of Las Vegas.

Alternative and Independent Festivals
Feminist Porn Awards
Toronto
www.goodforher.com
In 2006, the adult boutique Good for Her established the Feminist Porn Awards "because people don't know they have a choice when it comes to porn," according to former event organizer and Good for Her manager Chanelle Gallant. "There's a lot of bad porn out there," Gallant says, "but there is also some great porn being made by and for women. We wanted to recognize and celebrate the good porn makers as well as direct people to their work."[1]

PornfilmfestivalBerlin
Berlin
www.pornfilmfestival.de
Held every year in Berlin, but now with a second venue in Athens and soon to expand to Paris and Madrid, this is currently Europe's most important alternative porn festival and has something for everyone—from butch dykes to fans of feminist porn to transgender, gay, and straight people. The festival features extreme sexual experiments of

every kind as well as live shows that can make even the boldest blush.

Cum2Cut
Berlin

www.cum2cut.net

This competition takes place as part of Pornfilm festivalBerlin. A few days before Cum2Cut, the theme for a movie is announced along with other specifications, and directors and their crews have two days to shoot and edit.

CineKink NYC
New York

www.cinekink.com

As its name indicates, CineKink is indeed very kinky. In recent years, this festival has attracted not only new pornographic filmmakers but also a good number of talent scouts on the lookout for the next Martin Scorsese of porn. At the festival's conclusion, the winning films go on tour all over the United States.

Erotic Awards Events
London

www.erotic-awards.co.uk

This festival—a great excuse for a getaway to London, always a wonderful place to visit—is a rendezvous with the kinkiest that the United Kingdom has to offer. Every year, the best of the alternative and outrageous filmmakers get together, almost always in some quaint, picturesque spot.

Hump
Seattle

www.thestranger.com/hump

This alternative festival, sponsored by *The Stranger*, an alternative weekly newspaper in

Seattle, accepts erotica, animation, educational videos, kink—everything. A recent second-prize winner was a short film that starred a salt shaker and a napkin.

Good Vibrations Annual Independent Erotic Film Festival

San Francisco

www.gv-ixff.org/film

Good Vibes is a pioneer store that's focused on female pleasure since 1977. In 2006, they started the Good Vibrations Indie Erotic Film Festival at San Francisco's historic Castro Theatre. The competition became a full-fledged film festival in 2008 and now include international entries.

PORNOTOPIA

Albuquerque, New Mexico

www.selfservetoys.com

Imagine a world where erotic films don't offend, but arouse, where orgasms are real and filmmakers are independent. Self Serve periodically curates a collection of filmmakers who aren't afraid to keep it real when mainstream porn fails to satisfy. Pornotopia showcases sex on the big screen that is healthy, tender, raw, real, and beautiful.

A smorgasbord is a large, elaborate buffet of typical Swedish dishes. The Swedish word smörgåsbord is made up of the words for "sandwich" (smörgås) and "table" (bord), and the word smörgås in turn is a compound of smör (butter) and gås (goose). A smorgasbord is usually served at family gatherings or at festive events.

CHAPTER 9
A SMORGASBORD OF ADULT FILMS

FASTER, PUSSYCAT! KILL KILL!
Director: Russ Meyer (United States, 1965)

Turning your obsession into a way of life is certainly one of the best ways to cope with it. The director Russ Meyer, who acknowledged several times that he found making movies a sexual turn-on, took this idea a few steps further, not only earning a living (and quite a good one) from his outrageous movies, replete with wasp waists and huge breasts, but also making films that formed the basis of the sexploitation genre, which has lasted long enough to wow a whole new generation of moviegoers.

One of his most legendary films is *Faster, Pussycat! Kill Kill!* a car-chase orgy in which three she-devils on wheels take to the back roads of the Mojave Desert with misbehavior on their minds. The movie's opening leaves no room for doubt: "Ladies and gentlemen," a male voice-over intones, "welcome to violence, the word and the act. While violence cloaks itself in a plethora of disguises, its favorite mantle still remains . . . sex. Violence devours all it touches, its voracious appetite rarely fulfilled. Yet violence doesn't only destroy, it creates and molds as well. Let's examine closely, then, this dangerously evil creation,

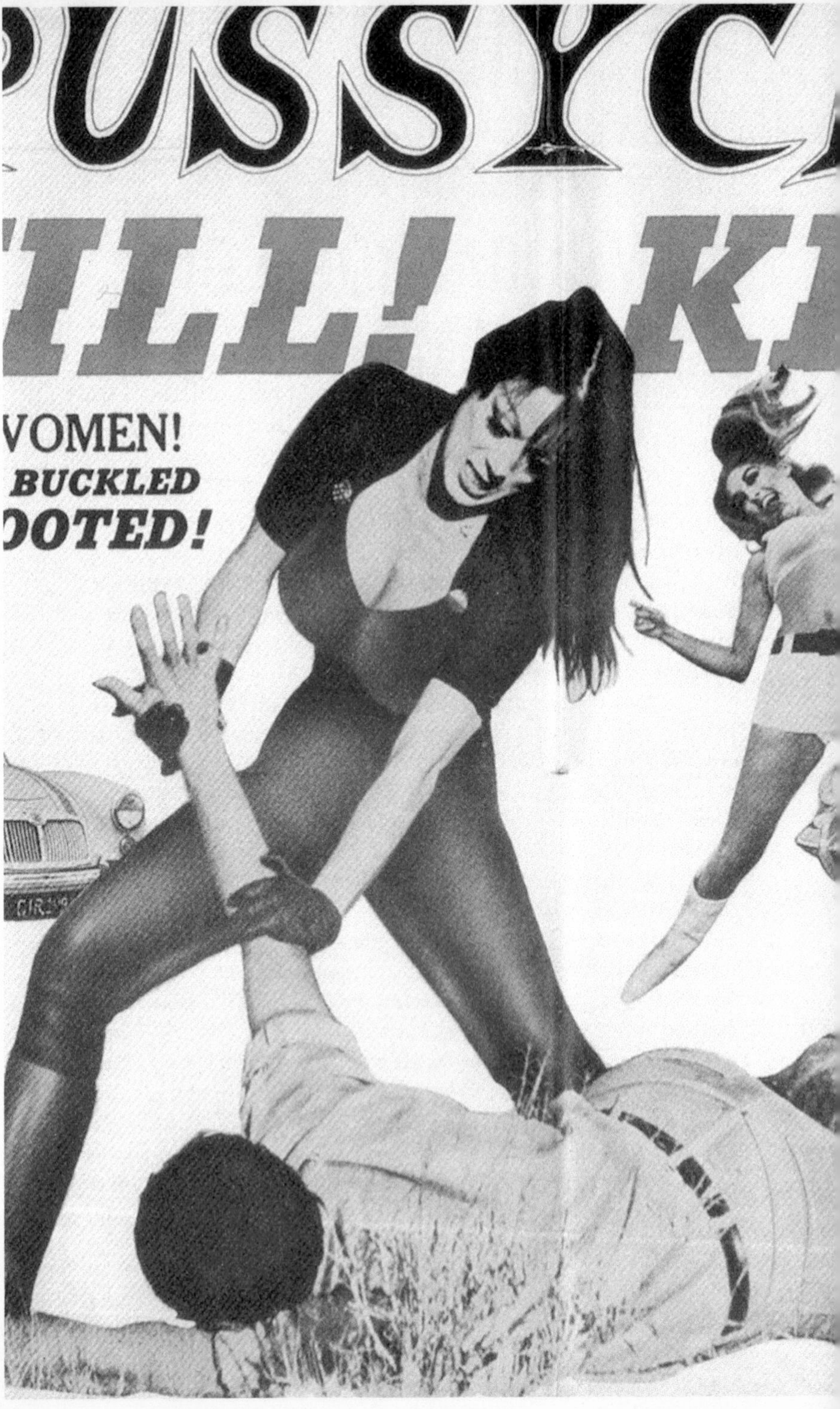

PUSSYC
ILL! KI
WOMEN!
BUCKLED
OOTED!

this new breed encased and contained within the supple skin of woman. The softness is there, the unmistakable smell of female, the surface shiny and silken, the body yielding yet wanton. But a word of caution—handle with care, and don't drop your guard. This rapacious new breed prowls both alone and in packs, operating at any level, any time, anywhere, and with anybody. Who are they? One might be your secretary, your doctor's receptionist . . . or a dancer in a go-go club!"

With that introduction out of the way—and with viewers duly warned about what lies ahead (a spoiler if ever there was one)—the three fearsome leading ladies enter the scene. First comes Varla, an evil brunette with exotic roots and an enormous rack (played by Tura Satana, in those days a starlet whose only previous film credit was for Billy Wilder's *Irma la Douce*). Then we have Rosie (played by Haji, another starlet and a former *Playboy* Playmate of the Month), a fierce, butchy Asian beauty. And finally there's Billie (Lori Williams, another *Playboy* alumna), a blonde as fearless as she is wild. The three of them are go-go dancers who drive around the desert looking for trouble in their sporty convertibles.

To start things off, they meet a young couple on the road and challenge the guy to a drag race. After the girls win, thanks to some outrageous cheating, they kill the guy and kidnap his innocent girlfriend, Linda. Their next stop is a gas station, where the attendant tells them about an old man living nearby who's hiding thousands of dollars in his house—the usual kind of information you get when you go for a fill-up. Varla decides that robbing the old guy is worth a side trip. The girls use their feminine wiles (and their voluptuous bodies) to settle into the house where the old man lives with his two sons, Tommy and The Vegetable (a muscled hulk who's not exactly the sharpest knife in the drawer). The girls' plan is to stay as long as it takes for them to make off with the old codger's money, and it never once occurs to them to throw in the towel, even though things aren't quite working out the way they were hoping.

If you can't find much meaning in this string of wicked deeds, don't worry. There really isn't any. You watch this Russ Meyer film to enjoy the action, including the moves of these women who get off on gratuitous violence and others' suffering—women who are evil in a way that, at least in the movies, only men had been before, girls with thick skin and plenty of cleavage—in what can be regarded as the first feminist revolution in world cinema.

LA DOLCE VITA
Director: Michael Lucas (United States, 2006)

The director Federico Fellini adored lusty, busty, voluptuous women, and he loved showing them in all their splendor, whether that meant Anita Ekberg wading into the Trevi Fountain in La Dolce Vita or Maria Antonietta Beluzzi as the buxom tobacconist in Amarcord. For that very reason, we don't know what this Italian director would have thought about the queer pornographic version of La Dolce Vita by the prolific producer and director Michael Lucas.[1]

Given the film's low budget, the action in Lucas's remake has to unfold not in Fellini's Rome but in present-day Manhattan, and specifically on the Upper West Side. There we meet Max Todd, played by Lucas himself, a journalist suffering from writer's block. Max goes looking for inspiration at one party after another, from the sketchiest parts of the city to elite fashion shows, and of course he scores here and there while also taking

176

in the action between other guys, all of whom have incredible bodies.

One of the film's most notable scenes was inspired by the episode in Fellini's film where Marcello Mastroianni and Anouk Aimee hire a prostitute for a three-way but then proceed to make mad passionate love themselves while the hired help sips coffee and listens to them from the next room. But in Michael Lucas's version, none of the three players (Lucas, Jason Ridge, and Derrick Hanson) stays outside. Instead, they have a phenomenal ménage à trois torrid enough to send the mercury spurting out of any thermometer that could have been used to record this threesome's heat.

Lucas's remake of *La Dolce Vita* preserves the spirit of the original, especially its tone of melancholy, the kind that descends when night falls and you're alone. Some critics have called Lucas's movie the saddest porn film ever made, a remark meant not as a criticism but as high praise.

The fact that the guys are handsome and sensual (just compare any one of the Lucas Entertainment actors with Ron Jeremy or other actors in mainstream porn), and that the art direction, the screenplay, and even the sound track are painstaking about details, makes this a perfect movie for women viewers, and it took prizes in all fourteen of the categories in which it was nominated at the 2007 GayVN Awards, the most important awards ceremony in gay adult films.

The film also includes a number of cameo performances by some well-known gay figures in nonsexual roles, such as Michael Musto of the *Village Voice* (he writes a gossip column called, aptly enough, "La Dolce Musto"), the transgender icon and New York nightlife hostess Amanda Lepore, and the female impressionist and fashion designer Kevin Aviance. It even has its own fountain scene to match the most famous scene in the original picture, this time with the actress Savana Samson. If Paris is worth a mass,[2] then aren't Rome and *La Dolce Vita*—and Manhattan, too, for that matter—reasons enough for a remake?

SUPERFREAK

Director: Shine Louise Houston (United States, 2006)

Shine Louise Houston is a veritable institution in the world of queer porn made by, with, and for women. She has her own company, Pink and White Productions, a B.F.A. in film from the San Francisco Art Institute, and a real talent for making girls come, whether they're on the screen or watching.

This director also has some intriguing thoughts about the adult film industry. She believes that if the industry exploits women, then it exploits men, too, and for the same reasons, so it's time to stop viewing women—those who are in the porn business and those who are not—as victims who should be pitied. Now that, I swear on Karl Marx, is revolutionary!

The performers in Houston's films are exclusively women (which is not to say that you won't see any penises—you will, but they'll be silicone), and they fuck on camera as if they were alone—without preconceptions, without restrictions, without looking at the camera, and without holding back.

Superfreak, Houston's second production, which won Best Dyke Sex Scene at the 2007 Feminist Porn Awards, tells the story of a girl (Madison Young) who is masturbating at home on her sofa, trying to blow off some sexual tension before going out for the evening, when she's possessed by the ghost of the R&B and funk singer Rick James (played by Houston herself in an engaging cameo). As a result, her hip, sensual attitude makes her the life of a party that gets totally out of hand and ends up as an orgy.

And here the humor ends, because when these girls fuck, they do it for real. To get things rolling, Young's character performs oral sex with a butchy girl who's packing a silicone dick, and the scene concludes with spectacular up-against-the-wall sex. After that comes oral sex in the kitchen (including water sports) and an impressively authentic, not to mention thorough, session of vaginal fist-fucking.

The movie is a nonstop parade of girls who have short fingernails, piercings, and tattoos, girls whose hair is dyed unreal colors, and girls who are having real orgasms (I was convinced, anyway, and I have a trained ear) in wild sex scenes that feature everything from anal sex to spanking to threesomes along with lots and lots of oral sex. And all this action is carried out by indie-style actresses who have a casual, no-fuss look but lots of dedication and plenty of smarts about what girls who like girls like to do with girls. In fact, *Superfreak* is one of the few movies I've ever seen where the actresses' eyes roll back—and the only one where you absolutely don't believe they're faking. The DVD includes some extras, including interviews with the director and the performers, outtakes, and a documentary about shooting the film, in which you can see all the work (and good vibes) that went on behind the camera.

DEEP THROAT
Director: Gerard Damiano (United States, 1972)

Along came the wild 1970s, and with them came the golden age of porn chic from the hand of the fabulous Gerard Damiano, a master of making films that went beyond the porn circuit and earned the

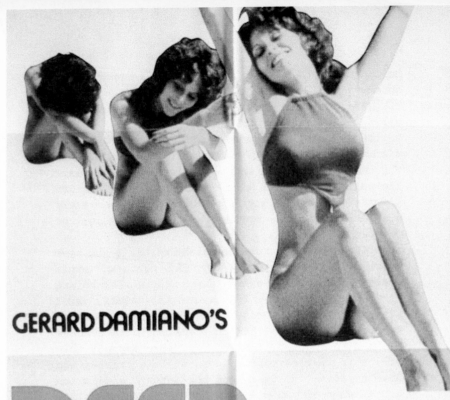

GERARD DAMIANO'S

DEEP THROAT

HOW FAR DOES A GIRL HAVE TO GO TO UNTANGLE HER TINGLE?

EASTMANCOLOR Ⓧ ADULTS ONLY

cult film status that got them shown in mainstream theaters and screened at mainstream festivals.

The first one out of the gate was *Deep Throat*, which tells the story of Linda (played by the legendary Linda Lovelace, also known as Linda Boreman), a woman who has never had an orgasm. After the film's first, rather arty scene, which lasts about five minutes and shows Linda driving to the house of her friend Helen (Dolly Sharp), things really pick up. Helen and Linda decide to put an end to Linda's anorgasmic state with some good sex, and they set up an orgy with a few friends, assuming that the earth will finally move for Linda. But not even this solves Linda's problem, so she goes to see Dr. Young (Harry Reems), a physician who collaborates with his nurse (Carol Connors) on some rather unusual diagnostic methods. He finally discovers Linda's problem—she has her clitoris at the back of her throat, a birth defect that Dr. Young discovers after several quite thorough examinations in which he takes a somewhat more than medical interest. To achieve her longed-for orgasms, Linda must master the art of fellatio, which is also what made Linda Lovelace one of the most famous fellators in the history of adult films.

The movie was shot and edited in just two weeks, at a cost of $25 million, about $1,200 of which went to Lovelace.[3] Today, nearly forty years later, *Deep Throat* has raked in more than $600 million and has been called the most profitable film in history.[4] Several remakes have already appeared (none as good as the original, unfortunately), and so has a documentary with the revealing title *Inside Deep Throat*, which uses compelling anecdotes to recount everything about the original movie, from the film shoot itself to the sad end of Linda Boreman[5] to the fierce opposition that came from the most conservative voices in American society when the film was released. This documentary includes interviews with famous directors and actors, such as Wes Craven, Francis Ford Coppola, and Warren Beatty, who describe how they felt about the movie the first time they saw it.

A curious footnote to the history of Damiano's film is that its title was also the nickname that two *Washington Post* reporters, Bob Woodward and Carl Bernstein, gave to an anonymous source of theirs who tore the lid off the Watergate scandal by implicating President Richard Nixon in the cover-up. He was William Mark Felt Sr., associate director of the FBI. The fact that Woodward and Bernstein gave him this nickname is a clear indication of *Deep Throat*'s cultural reach at the time of its release. The nickname Deep Throat is still commonly used to refer to someone who anonymously or indirectly feeds a journalist information.

9 SONGS

Director: Michael Winterbottom (United Kingdom, 2004)

When rumors began circulating that Michael Winterbottom, one of the icons of British independent cinema, was planning to make a sexually explicit film based on Michel Houllebecq's novel *Platform*, the high priests of the avant-garde thought their prayers had been answered—finally they would have a cultural alibi for jerking off, and they wouldn't be required to give up even a shred of their postmodernity. The first piece of bad news came just as the enthusiasm among fans and cinephiles was reaching fever pitch—Houllebecq already had his own plans for turning his novel into a movie, and so Winterbottom, who was still entertaining the idea of making an erotic film, had to go back to square one.

9 Songs was the result of this need to bring a sexually explicit story to the screen while ensuring

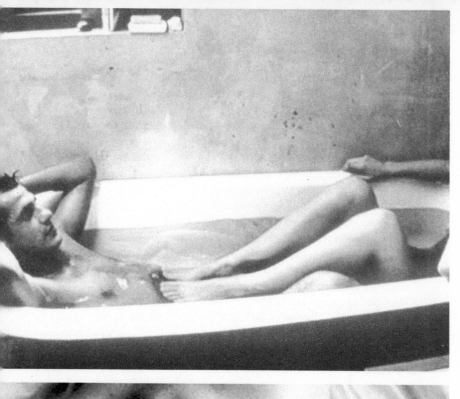
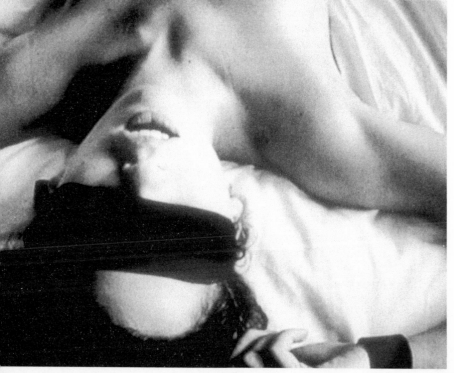

that it would have the look of a mainstream movie and the feel of an independent film. It's the story of Lisa, an American student spending a year in London, and Matt, the young Englishman who promptly becomes her lover. Winterbottom had everything he needed to make *9 Songs* an indie gem—unknown actors, digital equipment, a documentary style, and music made by and for young people.

The story goes more or less like this: Matt has always been fascinated by Antarctica and decides to visit the frozen continent. Once there, he begins to reminisce about his relationship with Lisa, in a series of flashbacks that blend with the wilderness of the South Pole, which makes Matt think of "claustrophobia and agoraphobia in one place—like two people in a bed." (Reading between the lines, we might translate this as male panic at the thought of commitment.)

From Lisa and Matt's first encounter, which takes place during a Black Rebel Motorcycle Club concert at London's Brixton Academy, the film's two leitmotifs, sex and music, punctuate a story that will end just before Christmas, when Lisa has to return home and her romp with the Londoner comes to an end.

The couple spends half the movie fucking (in the kitchen, in bed, anywhere and everywhere) and the other half going to what are mostly rock concerts. The sex scenes are very intense and realistic, and the two characters have great taste in music (the nine acts include Primal Scream, Franz Ferdinand, and the pianist Michael Nyman), but the plot is so loosely woven that the movie comes dangerously close to being a collection (though a very good one) of disconnected scenes.

Thankfully, every once in a while the directors of mainstream movies do need to show eroticism (as well as women characters who feel desire, feel love, and—why not?—feel like fucking). All of this helps to normalize sex on the screen. For that alone, we owe Michael Winterbottom a debt of heartfelt gratitude.

ARIA
Director: Andrew Blake (United States, 2001)

The American producer and director Andrew Blake (his real name is Paul Nevitt) is regarded as an innovator of adult films. His movies are all very much alike—he's one of those filmmakers who find a path and stick to it, never straying by so much as a centimeter.

So what is it that we see over and over in Blake's films? Gorgeous women, almost always in lesbian relationships—tall, sensual, sophisticated women modeling sumptuous undergarments, jewelry, garter belts, stockings, and spike heels, usually in fairly kinky settings. Although most of Blake's films are plotless erotic video clips that show these supermodels playing with themselves and each other, I still like the way he uses exquisite photography, elegant music (for a change), and beautifully designed sets to stage his male fantasies of lipstick lesbians. It's the polar opposite of gonzo.

Blake has his imitators, some of them quite good, such as Michael Ninn and Gregory Dark. Blake's

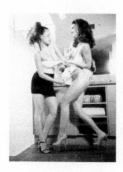 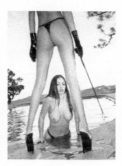 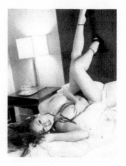

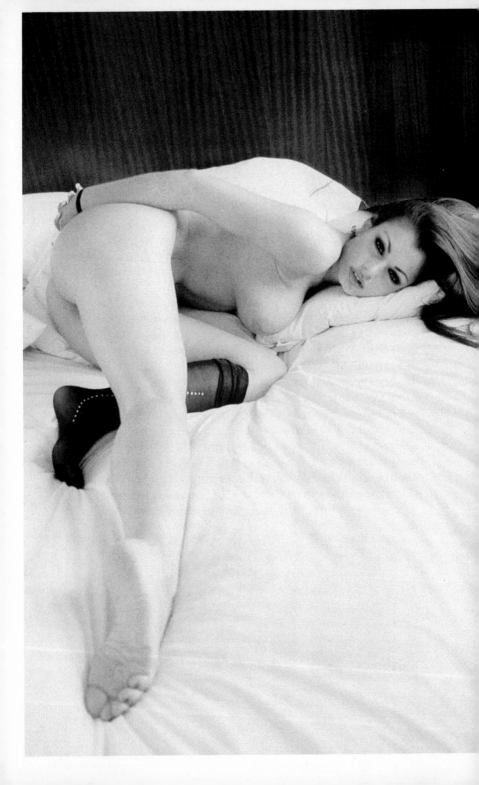

disciple and right-hand man, Nathan Strausse, recently struck out on his own to launch his own production company and make his first film, *Vignette*, which is somewhat more underground and alt than Blake's work.

I'm highlighting Blake's *Aria* here for several reasons. For one thing, there's the natural beauty of its star, Aria Giovanni, who in 2001 had just made her adult film debut. The film was conceived as an ode to Giovanni (born Cindy Renee Volk in Long Beach, California, to an Italian-Yugoslav father and a French-German-Irish-Indian mother). Giovanni is not a pornified adolescent but a voluptuous woman, almost an X-rated version of Monica Bellucci. And the rest of the girls in the cast are just as striking and could have stepped right out of a fashion magazine or a catalogue of fine lingerie like Agent Provocateur's. Another reason why I'm focusing on this particular Andrew Blake film is that it's one of his few to include a scene of heterosexual sex (in this case, between Sierra and Vince Voyeur), shot with the director's characteristic skill and taste.

EYES OF DESIRE
Director: Candida Royalle (United States, 1998)

Lisa (played by the ingénue Missy), an attractive photographer in the middle of a relationship crisis, goes to stay at the mountain chalet of some friends so she can take some time for herself and straighten out her life, as well as her relationship with her boyfriend, Jamie (Tony Tedeschi). As the result of a visit from a fun-loving friend (Sharon Mitchell), she discovers that the possibilities of the high-powered telescope in the living room go way beyond looking at the moon and the stars. She finds out that watching the neighbors fuck is much more entertaining than astronomy (and that voyeurism offers the additional advantage of being something she can indulge in day or night). Missy throws herself into her new hobby with real enthusiasm—and erotic outcomes. What she doesn't yet know is that in a supposedly vacant house across the way there is someone who is also looking at her, a mystery man who watches her exercising in the living room, working, and making passionate love with Jamie.

When she discovers this, she is prompted first by curiosity and then by lust to approach the mysterious house in search of the person who is spying on her. He turns out to be a gentleman named Daniel (Mickey G.), who admits that he can't take his eyes off her because he finds her so beautiful. She asks him indignantly what makes him think she's a loose woman, and she goes back to her borrowed house.

But now Lisa is no longer herself. In addition to her newfound enthusiasm for spying, she has discovered that it's also exciting to be spied on, and she fantasizes about the mystery man while she masturbates in the bathtub. That evening, knowing that Daniel is even more unsettled by her than he was before, she goes to the window and makes some provocative moves. Her telescopic Romeo responds by phoning her and asking her to undress and touch herself for him. After a moment's hesitation, she does, and when he invites her to come over, she doesn't think twice. She ends up in the arms of her admirer, and they make sweet hot love that concludes with a shared orgasm, many tender words, and a notice that the sequel to *Eyes of Desire* is coming soon.

I'm letting you know about this movie from Femme Productions because it may be the first film to stand out in the world of adult entertainment for having been written and directed by a woman and intended for a female audience. The director, Candida Royalle (discussed in more detail in chapter 7), had already made other movies, but none were as successful as *Eyes of Desire*, which continues to be a bestseller in the United States and elsewhere.

PINK PRISON
Director: Lisbeth Lynghøft (Denmark, 1999)

Pink Prison is a real oddity in auteurist pornographic film. First, it was co-produced with Zentropa, the company that belongs to Lars von Trier, a Danish director who usually makes mainstream movies. Second, it got such good reviews that it helped legalize porn in Norway (but not until March 12, 2006—the Norwegians were in no hurry). Third, its star, Katja Kean, also known as Katja K, has had one of the most unusual careers in adult films. She began working as a porn actress in 1997, at the age of twenty-nine, and three years later, at the height of her career and with only five movies behind her, she left to make mainstream movies, design lingerie, and give lectures on marketing. And, fourth, *Pink Prison*, together with *Constance* and *All About Anna*, belongs to the body of work produced by Innocent Pictures, and it's connected with the *Puzzy Power Manifesto* (see chapter 7), which calls for the prioritization of emotion and sensuality, realistic screenplays, the rejection of violence of any kind, and the elimination of gratuitous sex scenes in favor of a subtle buildup of desire.

Pink Prison tells the story of Mila (Katja K), a photojournalist working on a book of erotic photographs. She makes a bet with Yasia, her editor and lover, that she will succeed in getting into the penitentiary known as the Pink Prison to interview the warden, a mysterious man who has always avoided the press. If Mila wins the bet, she will

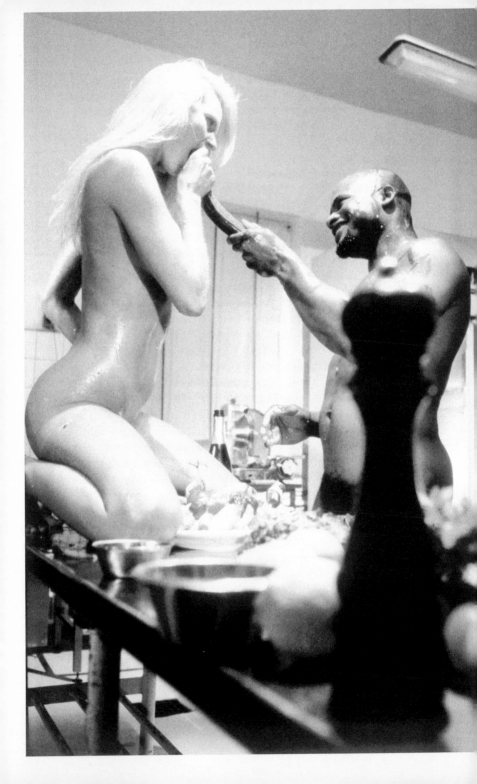

retain all rights to the book. If she loses, Yasia will be her guest on a weekend trip to Paris. Mila, a woman who fights for what she wants and is not to be messed with, is not discouraged when the normal channels fail to put her in touch with the warden. She determines to find an alternate route.

She finally manages to enter the prison by squeezing through an air duct. In the process, she becomes a voyeur, taking an active part in a series of erotic sequences that bring her closer and closer to her goal, which turns out to be utterly different from what she expected. One scene, remarkable for being so unusual in a heterosexually oriented film, involves anal sex between two men, which Mila watches through the grating in the air duct. Also remarkable, on aesthetic as well as erotic grounds, is the episode in which Mila, hiding in the showers, imagines herself being penetrated by three men. The entire film is marked by a quality of dreaminess (Mila has a marvelous sexual imagination), with the screen suffused in blue whenever the action takes place only in her mind.

Another remarkable aspect of the film is its screenplay, which greatly transcends the classic pornographic plot trajectory (which is usually just an excuse for linking one sex scene to the next). *Pink Prison* is interesting enough and good enough to watch all the way through, and not necessarily with masturbation in mind.

THE DEVIL IN MISS JONES
Director: Gerard Damiano (United States, 1973)

It's not particularly unusual for a pornographic movie to start out with a bathtub scene, as any fan of the genre knows. If the main character is in the tub because she wants to slit her wrists, well, that's different. But so begins *The Devil in*

Miss Jones, Gerard Damiano's second successful film after the boom he had set off the year before with *Deep Throat*.

The heroine, Justine Jones, is played by the legendary Georgina Spelvin, virtually a beginner and, in 1973, pushing forty, an age when most porn actresses have retired. Fed up with her boring, solitary, virginal existence, Miss Jones kills herself. Her only remaining consolation is the possibility of going to heaven after she's dead. But things don't work out that way. Although she has lived a life free of sin, her suicide bars her from heaven, and so she's directed to limbo, the worst place a spirit can end up. Terrified by the turn things have taken, Miss Jones begs for a little more time on earth. Her wish is granted, on one condition—that she allow herself to be led along the lustful ways of the flesh by a mysterious guide played by Harry Reems (called The Teacher) so she can finally earn a place in hell as a libertine.

From the moment Miss Jones accepts this proposition, she is swept into a frenetic succession of sex acts of every kind and quantity. And from the beginning, her mentor shows her that he has no time for little girls. He carries out Justine's anal defloration brutally, with a dildo, but Justine, far from being intimidated by this drastic initiation, is dying of curiosity and wants more. Her mentor's penis becomes her playmate. Through it she learns about all the things of which she knew nothing in her previous life, and she reveres it as a phallic totem. Now nothing is out of bounds. She tries one-to-one lesbianism (with the actress Judith Hamilton, also her lover in real life) as well as lesbian sex in orgies that include men, where she participates in a landmark two-mouth blow job. She also masturbates with various types of fruits and vegetables and even, in a scene that has become iconic, turns an actual snake to sexual purposes. But the film's most affecting moment is certainly when Miss Jones is seen again in the same bathtub where, days before, she took her own life. Now, in a desperate attempt to cling to life, she masturbates (to the accompaniment of a sound track whose epic strains seem to have been borrowed from a western), only to find herself quickly dragged down to hell as just punishment for her sins.

The Devil in Miss Jones was so successful, both within and outside the porn world, that six sequels were made, each one worse than the one before, and not one as good as the original.

CONTES IMMORAUX
Director: Walerian Borowczyk (France, 1974)

Very few directors in the world of art films and experimental filmmaking have told erotic stories the way Walerian Borowczyk (1923–2006) has done. This painter, graphic artist, writer, and director of Polish films is also the director of the fantastic *Contes Immoraux*.

The film wallows in the pleasures of sin, looking at sexuality from the darkest, most enthralling angles to confuse (and unsettle) the viewer, thanks to some impressive visual effects that are very hard to find in other films of this genre, and that are found here partly because of the importance this director places on historical accuracy, set design, and art direction.

The "immoral stories" are four vignettes that follow a prologue, presented in the form of title cards like the ones in a silent film, which fills us in on the background of the scenic tableaux we are about to see. A bit of reading, and off we go into the thick of things.

The first of the stories, *La Marée* (based on a

short story by the noted French writer André Pierre de Mandiargues, who also wrote the screenplay), shows us a young man of twenty cunningly explaining the movement of the tides as a way of showing his cousin, a young girl inexperienced in these matters, how to perform a blow job.

The second story, *Thérèse Philosophe*, is a tale of autoeroticism in which an extremely pious young woman uses her restless hands, and two cucumbers, to deal with the excitement provoked in her by candelabras and other liturgical knickknacks. After listening to her recite what has to be the most erotic Lord's Prayer ever, you're going to have trouble going to church ever again for a wedding, a baptism, or anything else without recalling that sensual scene. You've been warned.

The third story, *Erzsébet Bathory*, is probably the most famous of the group, partly because of its star, a designer and perfumer best known as her father's daughter—Paloma Picasso, who plays the sadistic Transylvanian aristocrat of the title, nicknamed the Bloody Duchess for her habit of bathing in the blood of virgins in her quest for eternal youth. The scene in which several dozen young ladies take a shower, only to be murdered later, in the midst of a frenzied ball, is both so beautiful and so disquieting that it gives you the chills.

To conclude the film, Borowczyk, in *Lucrezia Borgia*, lets himself fantasize about the orgies of Italy's most powerful family. In a story filled with religious imagery, where sex scenes alternate with messages of intense religiosity, the title character gives herself to her father, Pope Alexander VI, and to her brother, Cardinal Cesare Borgia.

Ultimately, like all Borowczyk's other works, *Contes Immoraux* is marked by a surprising aesthetic perfection. It is equally interesting as a conceptual work and as one that is erotically charged.

L'AMANT/THE LOVER

Director: Jean-Jacques Annaud (France/United Kingdom, 1992)

The Lover is based on the autobiographical novel of the same title by Marguerite Duras, one of my favorite writers. This movie, filled with moments of passion, also includes one of my favorite sex scenes, although it's nowhere near being an X-rated film.

It presents the love story of a poor white fifteen-year-old girl (played by Jane March) and a rich, attractive Chinese businessman (Tony Leung Ka Fai) in the Vietnam of the late 1920s, when the country was under French occupation. From the moment the businessman spots the girl on the Mekong River ferry—with painted lips, in a threadbare dress and a hat whose ribbon is trailing in the wind, dressed up like a woman without yet being one—he can't help feeling attracted to her, and he offers her a ride to Saigon in his chauffeured car.

Their relationship grows stronger as they spend time together, with the businessman accompanying the girl from school to the dormitory where she sleeps, until one afternoon they end up in bed, where they make love sweetly, almost nostalgically—and, interestingly, it's the girl who makes the first move. This scene, like the film's other sex scenes, was shot with the craftsmanship and elegance that mark Annaud's work, letting us see how beautifully sex can be shown on the screen if that is a director's intention.

The relationship takes a tragic turn when other people get involved. The girl's attempt to introduce her lover to her family is a disaster—her coarse, racist brothers and her mother get drunk, ignoring and practically insulting him, and an incident with incestuous overtones involving her older brother makes her Asian lover wildly jealous. As for the

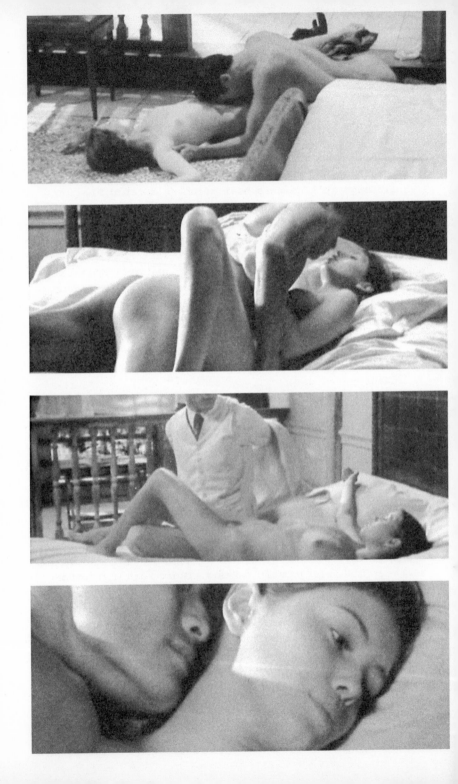

mother, the generosity of her daughter's lover, and her own poverty and neediness, cause her just to look the other way most of the time.

L'Amant, the novel on which this movie is based, won the Prix Goncourt in 1984, the finishing touch to the long and prolific literary career of Marguerite Duras. As a novelist, she was one of the twentieth century's most controversial, in her written work as well as in her personal life. The fact that toward the end of her life she took up with a man thirty years her junior may have had something to do with the controversy. In 1996, Duras was buried in Paris, in the cemetery at Montparnasse, but she continues to inspire young people with the power and passion of her words.

BELLADONNA'S FUCKING GIRLS AGAIN
Director: Belladonna (United States, 2005)

Belladonna may be one of the most highly sexed women on the face of the earth. She likes her sex rough, dirty, and without taboos or restrictions of any kind (as long as it's consensual and between adults, of course). In the beginning, her production company, Belladonna Entertainment, produced only rough, high-voltage lesbian porn but is now making some of the hardest-core films in adult entertainment today. Anal sex (Belladonna adores it, having lost her anal virginity on camera, and she says she enjoyed it even the first time), extreme fetishism, spanking, more or less soft S&M, and transgender sex are never in short supply in films by Belladonna, who is also well known for having been Nacho Vidal's real-life girlfriend.

It's interesting that one of the most controversial movies ever to come out of her production company was Belladonna's Fucking Girls Again, an exclusively lesbian film that the actress

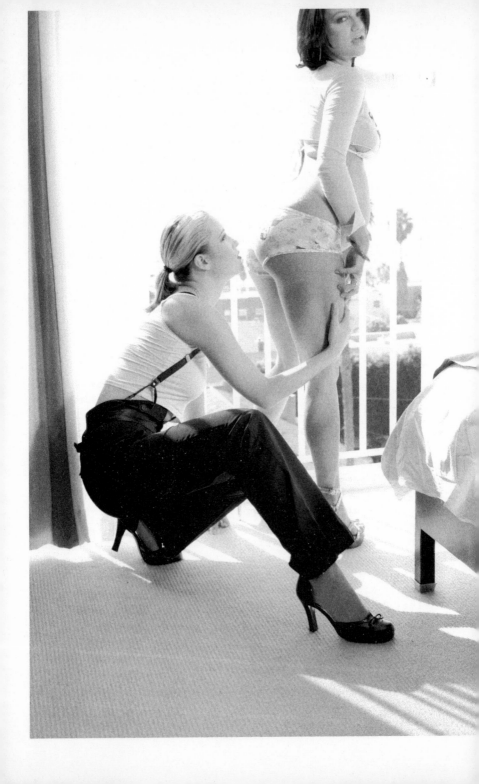

and director shot when she was six or seven months pregnant. It seems that the sight of a big-bellied Belladonna having sex on the camera was enough to scandalize even the fans of porn's crudest subgenre. In the first scene, Belladonna persuades her girlfriend, the actress Jackie Moore, to do a sexy striptease for her. Meanwhile, Belladonna polishes a pair of high-top black boots and a harness outfitted with a big black dildo with which she attempts to dominate Jackie in every possible way. But Belladonna also gets a taste of her own medicine when Jackie penetrates her with the dildo by the light of the setting sun.

The next segment features two Asian-looking girls, Lucy Lee and Nautica Thorn. Belladonna breaks out a regular showcase of sex toys, and the two girls put them to good use. Vibrators, glass dildos, and anal beads in all sizes and colors abound in a scene where the oral sex and the chemistry between the girls are simply stunning.

A little later Belladonna is back, this time with the actress Kimberly Kane in a nice sunny hotel room. First Kimberly, wearing an elegant pair of men's formal pants with suspenders, watches in fascination as Belladonna plays with herself. Then she joins in to share kisses and vibrators, anal sex, and a lot of saliva.

The next stop is what appears to be a room in a student dormitory, with twin beds made up with red sheets on which Barbara Summer is giving Kat a lesson in tonguing. The scene concludes with a red-hot sex scene in which they show how many inches of a vibrator they can insert anally.

And in the final scene, where Belladonna looks about nine months pregnant, she has what is probably the roughest sex of the whole movie, in a bathroom with Melissa, a French blonde with pretty blue eyes. The sex is wild and very very hot, with hints of domination, and it culminates with the blonde's head being shoved into the washbasin.

SHORTBUS
Director: John Cameron Mitchell (United States, 2006)

Shortbus is the name of a no-holds-barred sex club in present-day New York where the sex is of a piece with avant-garde music and art. It's the spot where several New Yorkers' lives converge, lives as different as they are fundamentally alike. We have the punk dominatrix Severin; James and Jamie, a gay couple in crisis looking for the ideal man to make a threesome (Jamie, as it happens, is still hung up on his past as a child actor in a television series); and Sofia, a sexually frustrated sex therapist married to Rob.

The characters' stories begin to come together when James and Jamie decide they'll try therapy to deal with their relationship problems. That's how they meet their sex therapist, Sofia, who has a secret that's ironic, to say the least, in view of her profession—she has never had an orgasm. James and Jamie decide to do something about it. They take her to Shortbus, with the intention of putting an end to her problem. They believe that at Shortbus, where nothing is prohibited, something will stimulate her enough to make her come. And there she meets Severin, a dominatrix for hire whose sexuality is so intense that her character might almost be regarded as antagonistic, but Severin becomes Sofia's friend and confidante.

The club's master of ceremonies, a drag performer of sorts named Justin Bond, defines Shortbus as a place for pleasure and exchange, a place where you can just watch or go ahead and take part in orgies and threesomes or have sex by yourself or do S&M—

200

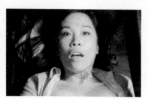 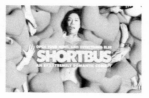 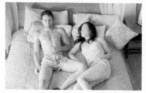

any and every form of sexual expression is welcome at Shortbus. "It's like the sixties, but with less hope," Justin says, straddling the line between irony and melancholy. In reality, though, Shortbus is also an assembly of lonely hearts looking for something like love.

The life-affirming atmosphere (with sex-positivity as one of its effects) of post-9/11 New York is perfectly sketched in this social and generational portrait by John Cameron Mitchell (who also directed *Hedwig and the Angry Inch*, one of the most impressive musicals since *The Rocky Horror Picture Show*). *Shortbus* does include explicit sex scenes (but no medical shots), whose sole purpose is to portray human relationships fully and honestly. Made with a budget that was negligible even by the standards of independent films, it used a cast of professional actors as well as amateurs found through newspaper and Internet ads.

CHEMISTRY, VOLUMES 1–4
Director: Tristan Taormino (United States, 2006–2008)

Tristan Taormino is a writer, a columnist, a director of adult films, and a sex educator. She has written several books and has a fantastic website (www.puckerup.com) whose slogan is "smart sexy anal kinky fun," and that's what her site is all about. The same spirit imbues the name of her company, Smart Ass Productions. Taormino defines her work as a reaction against the porn of recent decades. "Through my workshops and other travels," she says,

"I've had the opportunity to talk to hundreds of different people. Plenty of men and women tell me that they love all-sex and gonzo videos, but could do without some of the elements of the most popular titles in those genres. Plus, they're tired of seeing videos where the women either don't come or their orgasms are clearly fake. That's where Smart Ass Productions comes in. No outrageous stunts. No degradation. Instead, the focus is on fresh and accessible performers, hot, spontaneous sex, real chemistry and real orgasms for everyone."[6]

The concept behind the *Chemistry* series, as described in the film's publicity materials, is "7 Stars. 1 House. 36 Hours. No Script. No Schedule. Just Sex The Way They Want It." It's something like the *Big Brother* reality TV series. In *Chemistry 1*, for example, Taormino simply watches Dana DeArmond, Jack Lawrence, Kurt Lockwood, Marie Luv, Mr. Marcus, Mika Tan, and Taryn Thomas interact. She interviews them and introduces them to us, and she also gives us another perspective with the "perv cam," a camera without an operator that the actors speak to individually, using it as a type of private confessional.

What Taormino has staged is the popular fantasy of going away for the weekend to a house with a group of friends and, once locked inside, giving free rein to fantasies as well as to nonstop orgiastic sex, with everybody doing whatever they want with whomever they want.

A big reason why the *Chemistry* series works as well as it does is that Taormino gives us a cast of actors who have distinct personalities and something to say. They're not just bodies fucking like mad. They let the viewer in on their feelings and fantasies, and as a result we get to know them and can understand how the chemistry among them develops (hence the title of the series).

I like *Chemistry* because of its refreshing

realism, and because of the fact that what's on the screen is believable. The performers aren't perceived as mere actors but as ordinary people who happen to be uninhibited and unafraid to express and share their sexuality. And we're not bored by the predictable porn formula of a blow job and three positions, followed by the money shot. Instead, the sex takes place without rules, as people feel like having sex in the moment.

Chemistry has won quite a few awards at mainstream and alternative porn festivals. With her simple but beautifully executed idea, Taormino has herself a hit.

DESTRICTED

Directors: Marina Abramovic, Matthew Barney, Marco Brambilla, Larry Clark, Gaspar Noé, Richard Prince, Sam Taylor-Wood (United States, 2006)

If I start by saying that *Destricted* is a sexually explicit film that has won prizes at Sundance and Cannes as well as at film festivals in Edinburgh and Amsterdam, you'll realize right away what an unconventional work it is. When I tell you that it had a weeklong screening at the Tate Modern, you'll begin to understand the magnitude of this project, and if I tell you who had a hand in it—names like Larry Clark, Matthew Barney, and the photographer and video artist Sam Taylor-Wood, among others—you'll see that we're talking more about a work of art than a work of pornography, because *Destricted* is brimming with art, from the title (a play on the word "restricted") to the last frame.

Sam Taylor-Wood, for example, conceived of erotica in terms of filming (flawlessly, needless to say) many long minutes of a man masturbating after having journeyed to dusty Death Valley, the place that gives her short its title, in a sequence that

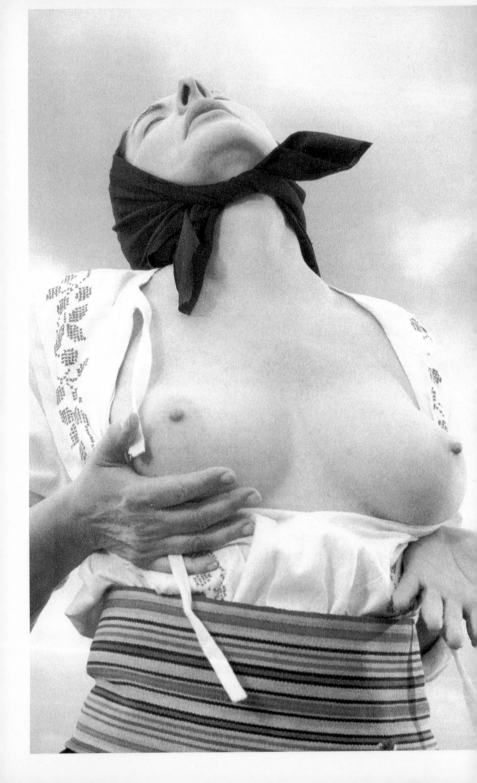

leaves both the man and the viewer in a state of near exhaustion. By contrast, Marco Brambilla needed no more than three minutes to show us his vision of sex in the shortest of these shorts, *Sync*, which consists of juxtaposed pornographic images flashed across the screen for less than a second, creating a sense of unease and disorientation.

Matthew Barney's piece, *Hoist*, depicts the peculiar relationship between a man and a Caterpillar tractor that has undergone some unusual mutations. This piece is as interesting to watch as it is difficult to associate with any form of eroticism as we know it.

Gaspar Noé, who in his film *Irréversible* staged one of the most disturbing scenes in all of cinema—the nine-minute-long rape of Alex (Monica Bellucci) by a character known only as The Tapeworm (Jo Prestia)—presents *We Fuck Alone*, an explicit masturbation scene showing a childish-looking girl who touches herself with some help from her teddy bear while watching a pornographic movie as a punkish-looking guy has his way, at gunpoint, with a blow-up doll.

Finally, I have to mention *Impaled*, Larry Clark's contribution. Clark, an avowed sex addict, has never hesitated to show explicit sex in his films about adolescents. In his thirty-minute piece, we watch as he interviews several young indie-looking guys (they could all be performers in any of his movies) for what ends up being a porn film that culminates in a full-out cumshot.

I like *Destricted* because it's bold, provocative, aesthetically pleasing, and conceptually quite interesting, and because it forced the generally rather uptight little world of contemporary conceptual art to take the risk of seeing sex as just one among many kinds of expression.

LE SEXE QUI PARLE
Director: Claude Mulot (France, 1975)

This movie deserves a stop on our tour of sexually explicit films because it's the only one with a character who literally gives voice to what her cunt is feeling. That character is Joelle, a thirtysomething Parisian and the owner of a talking vagina (a phenomenon sure to strike more fear into the hearts of men than the *vagina dentata* of folklore).

The voice of Joelle's cunt incites her to all manner of sex acts. Her labia minora are ironic, rude, and irreverent, and they're not afraid to say all the things their big sisters have to keep quiet about. They even call Joelle's husband, Eric, an imbecile, a good-for-nothing, a lousy lay, and other choice epithets whenever the opportunity arises. And the remarks of Joelle's vagina—which has obviously been left high and dry by the inept Eric—lead Joelle to surprise her coworkers with blow jobs, touch herself in front of Eric's friends, and seek out furtive experiences of all kinds. Joelle's talking cunt even has its own cinematic point of view, conveyed through a recurring visual effect that shows us not only *what* the vagina sees (genitals, faces, and so forth) but also *how* the vagina sees, thanks to an overlay in the shape of a vertically oriented almond. This film is a mix, rare in adult films, of boldness, strangeness, modernity, and especially humor.

When Eric realizes that his wife's new mouth has no intention of keeping quiet, he decides that the two of them—his wife and her second mouth (or, depending on how you look at it, the three of them: his wife, her talking labia, and her talking vagina)—should consult a woman psychoanalyst and get to the bottom of what certainly has to be the strange, pathological result of some sexual trauma.

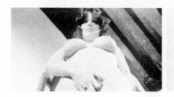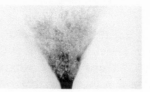

Naturally, the appointment doesn't resolve a thing, and it ends in sex. But then, at a huge press conference, the psychoanalyst reveals the existence of the talking vagina and the media go crazy, forcing Eric and Joelle to flee the city.

On their way out of town, they spend the night in a hotel, the setting for one of the best scenes in the movie. While Joelle is asleep, her cunt and Eric, both of them hoping to bring about some kind of détente, have a conversation in which the vagina tells Eric what its sex life was like before Eric, and about how good things used to be. The vagina leaves no room for doubt that there is no hope of reaching an understanding with a lover as boring as Eric. At this point, Eric decides to give the so-called battle of the sexes its full meaning—attempting to shut Joelle's second mouth up, he smothers it by shoving his penis inside.

DEBBIE DOES DALLAS
Director: Jim Clark (United States, 1978)

Debbie, the head cheerleader at her high school, has been invited to join the cheerleading squad of a professional football team in Dallas, but her parents have absolutely forbidden her to go. Nothing can stop little Debbie, though. She convinces several of her fellow cheerleaders to take the trip with her, and she promises that they'll all become famous. But none of them have the money to go to Dallas, as they realize when it becomes clear that crappy jobs in hamburger joints and retail stores won't even earn them a livable wage, much less money for little jaunts.

Things start to change when Mr. Greenfield, Debbie's boss at the sporting goods store where she works, offers Debbie ten dollars if she'll show him her boobs, and another ten if she'll let him touch them, and another ten on top of that if she'll let him lick them. And so the Dallas cheerleading hopeful quickly learns that there are other and faster ways for a girl to make some cold hard cash than actually going to bed with somebody and losing her precious virginity. Pretty soon the whole squad is working toward its financial goals by engaging in sexual transactions that range from hand jobs to threesomes, and from blow jobs to anal sex. One airhead even manages to misplace her virginity.

But Debbie's boss is getting tired of always hearing her say no whenever he asks her to let him penetrate her. Finally he makes her an offer she can't refuse—if she gives him her virginity, he'll not only pay her way to Dallas, he'll pay for all her friends to go, too.

In the scene that serves as the movie's grand finale, Debbie is dressed as a cheerleader for the Dallas football team, and Mr. Greenfield is dressed as the team's captain. They lick each other all over and have oral sex, and then Debbie and Mr. Greenfield have intercourse, first with Debbie on top and then in the missionary position. Just before the credits roll, the words "Touchdown for Mr. Greenfield" and "Score one for Debbie" appear on the screen, followed by the word "Next."

And this, more or less, is the plot of the first movie to star the newcomer Bambi Woods—an adaptation of the high school comedy genre, and a high-voltage look at the world of cheerleaders. But it had to be filmed on a university campus, and so the producers had no qualms about lying when the time came to obtain the necessary permits. Officials at the State University of New York at Stony Brook were so flattered that these filmmakers wanted to immortalize their school that they didn't hesitate to give them free access, and they even played themselves in one scene. But what the producers conveniently forgot to tell them was that this was a pornographic movie, and when the truth came out, the officials were fired.[7]

This story about the adventures of Debbie and her friends was successful beyond anyone's wildest expectations. The movie earned millions of dollars as well as the honor of becoming the best-selling pornographic movie of the 1980s—and that's saying something.

CINCO HISTORIAS PARA ELLAS/FIVE HOT STORIES FOR HER

Director: Erika Lust (Spain, 2007)

It's really hard to comment on your own work without giving way to self-satisfaction or, at the other extreme, excessively harsh self-criticism, so this summary was the hardest one for me to write in the whole book.

When I decided to get myself mixed up in the grand adventure of directing an adult film, my basic intention was to make the kind of movie that women like me wanted to see but weren't finding anywhere— a sexually explicit film for women, couples, or men who wanted more from porn than a succession of medical shots, a film for people who wanted porn

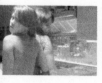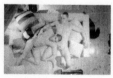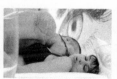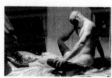

that had a sense of humor, porn with elegance, style, and respect for female characters.

These are the premises that led to *Five Hot Stories for Her*, the first movie from my Lust Films production company, which was coproduced with Thagson Women. It's a compilation of five modern, cosmopolitan, explicit shorts about sex.

Something About Nadia is a tale of seduction and desire that revolves around the title character (played by Sandra G), a mysterious, very attractive lesbian.

FuckYouCarlos.com tells the story of Sonia's sexy, very funny revenge against her serially unfaithful husband, Carlos, a soccer player. To get back at him, she films her world-class three-way with a couple of his teammates and then puts the footage up on the Internet.

Married with Children begins with a look at Frank and Rita, a couple who appear to have fallen into the routine boredom of living together. Their sex life seems to have vanished in the rush of daily chores, children, and work, but the surprising truth that we discover at the end of this short shows us the couple's more sensual side.

The Good Girl explores one of porn's most typical fantasies—the one about the delivery guy who shows up at the front door of a woman who freely surrenders to him.

In *Breakup Sex*, we investigate the phenomenon named in the title, those shared orgasms that we scratch out at the end of a relationship, denying the evidence that it's over, and—perhaps because we actually do understand this truth—giving ourselves with all the passion we have in us.

Five Hot Stories for Her was named best screenplay at the Festival de Cine Erótico (Barcelona 2007), best film for women at the Erotic E-line Awards (Berlin, 2007), and best film of the

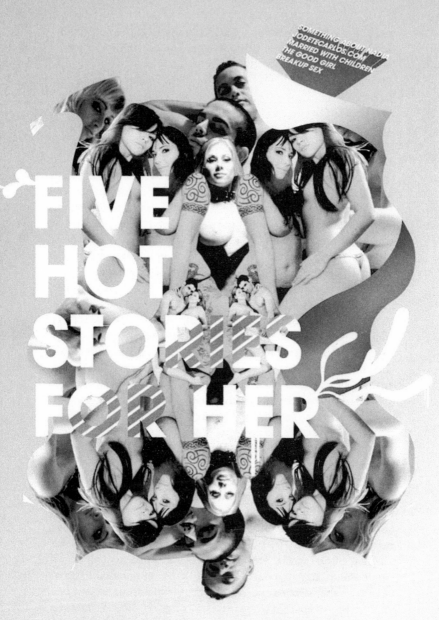

year at the Feminist Porn Awards (Toronto, 2008) and received an honorable mention at the CineKink Festival (New York, 2008).

SECRETARY

Director: Steven Shainberg (United States, 2002)

When Lee Holloway (Maggie Gyllenhaal) shows up at the law office of E. Edward Grey (James Spader) and applies for a secretarial position, nothing could convince you that she will ever get this or any other job. Her résumé would make even the most jaded human resources manager weep tears of blood. She has never worked a day in her life, she comes from a dysfunctional family, she has just been discharged from a psychiatric hospital, and she's a self-cutter.

Improbable though it seems, Mr. Grey hires Lee, and she begins her professional life by performing routine tasks like filing, making coffee, and feeding letters through a postage machine. But, little by little, something that could be sensed at the beginning becomes more and more obvious—what Mr. Grey really needs is not a secretary but a submissive female, and what Lee really needs is not a job but a domineering male.

Lee needs to keep satisfying Mr. Grey's expectations, and he needs to keep setting the bar higher and higher in their games of consensual humiliation, and so their relationship gradually moves farther and farther away from the realm of work. The two of them have written the rules for this sexual game they're playing, which no one else can understand. And despite the crudeness of some scenes, the movie communicates a curious aura of tenderness throughout, a notion of sadomasochistic relationships that is difficult to grasp—the notion of love wrapped in pain. Of course Lee's family and loved ones, including an insufferable pseudo

212

boyfriend, try to make her quit her job and leave her boss, lover, and master. But, luckily or unluckily, she has already discovered what love is and is unwilling to give it up, no matter what. An offbeat, very black sense of humor permeates the film and makes *Secretary* one of the darkest, most politically incorrect romantic comedies ever made, light years from any Hollywood spawn starring the likes of Cameron Diaz.

I'm discussing this movie in the company of my favorite erotic films not because of its pornographic scenes (which are nonexistent) or its erotic scenes (also few in number, though there is a spanking scene that should go down in history) but because of the intensity of what this film suggests but never once shows. One of the film's strong points is its cast. The role of E. Edward Grey seems made to order for James Spader, with his expressive features and his ability to find an unusual comic aspect in the part, and Maggie Gyllenhaal is perfect as the timid, homely, self-destructive girl transformed into a personification of wild sensuality. Although *Secretary* won a number of prizes at independent festivals, reviewers endlessly criticized the film because they did not understand how it could start out with a European sensibility but have a happy ending of the most purely American kind.

BEHIND THE GREEN DOOR
Directors: James and Artie Mitchell (United States, 1973)

Since we've already talked about some other 1970s cult movies, we can't fail to mention *Behind the Green Door*, a film by the Mitchell Brothers based on a World War II-era urban myth that warned about the dangers of girls stopping off at roadhouses, only to be abducted, drugged, and forced to take part in spectacular orgies in front of an audience.

Something very much like that is what happens to this film's main character, played by Marilyn Chambers, whose face was already well known because of her involvement in an advertising campaign for the brand of soap powder called Ivory Snow, whose slogan was "99 and 44/100% Pure." The Mitchell Brothers capitalized on her face recognition by billing her as the "99 and 44/100% pure" girl. Her innocent, virginal look was largely responsible for her success, and she became an adult film legend on a par with Traci Lords and Linda Lovelace herself.[8]

Behind the Green Door begins with two truck drivers walking into a roadside bar. The owner asks them what they know about some abductions of young women, and one of the drivers admits having witnessed one such event. He decides to tell his story, and listening at a neighboring table is Gloria (Marilyn Chambers), looking sad and drinking a beer. Later she's abducted herself and taken off to a mysterious place where anything can happen.

After being given drugs and a relaxing massage, Gloria is led to a stage where she sees a masked man and six other women. This is a show, and its only purpose is to give her every conceivable kind of pleasure. The six women get down to business, soon to be followed by members of the audience (including a few African American actors, which was quite revolutionary at the time, since Chambers was a white woman), and they all join in a final, massive orgy.

Slow-motion on-camera ejaculations, the orgy, mimes and clowns, and scenes with trapezes as well as other kinds of circus paraphernalia made *Behind the Green Door* a true artistic experiment, since until this time the Mitchell Brothers had produced only short films. The directors' fondness for the psychedelic, aesthetic, and LSD had a strong influence on how they handled imagery in the film, which plays with stroboscopic effects, blurry and out-of-focus shots, colored filters, and other visual effects seldom used in pornographic movies. Artie Mitchell's weakness for narcotics also played a part in his unfortunate end, and his brother Jim shot him to death after a heated argument.[9]

EAST SIDE STORY
Director: Vena Virago (United States, 2007)

Vena Virago, an alternative artist from Los Angeles, is known for her drawings, graffiti, paintings, and art installations. When she started out as a porn director, it was because she wanted to combine her personal aesthetic and her artistic vision with her passion for adult films, and so she joined the directors of Vivid-Alt, the division of Vivid Entertainment headed by Eon McKai.

Her first film for Vivid-Alt was *East Side Story*, a tale that takes us into the heart of East Los Angeles, where we meet an eclectic group of characters. They tell us, reality-style, about their sexual histories, and then we watch them fuck as elements in a series of art installations created by Virago. The film has been described as

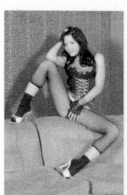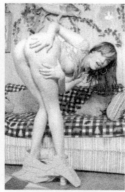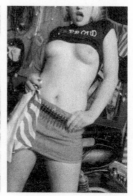

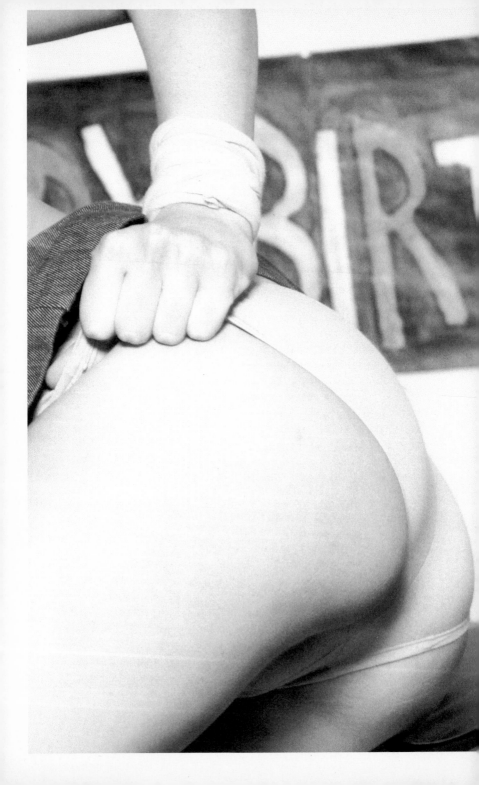

"part documentary, part abstract painting, and all-out multicultural hardcore."[10]

The results are quite interesting, and if you like extras, you'll find plenty of them on the DVD, including an almost hour-long "making of" feature that will give you a truly intimate look at the performers if you feel you still don't know them after watching the film itself. If you're curious about the alt guys and girls performing in adult movies—in this case, Rebeca Linares, Dana DeArmond, Michelle Aston, Lexi Bardot, Roxy DeVille, Page Morgan, Dino Bravo, Tyler Knight, and Alex Gonz— then this is a great opportunity to see them in their element.

Also worth noting is the film's sound track, with music by the Selectrons, the Harvey Cartel, Travi Soul, and Babyhans.

AFRODITE SUPERSTAR

Director: Venus Hottentot (United States, 2007)

Generally speaking, there's more diversity and multiculturalism in porn than in any other film genre because porn is a friendly, teeming playground for people of all races and all social circumstances. But African American audiences in the United States want their own adult films, so Femme Chocolat, the "ebony" division of Candida Royalle's Femme Productions, came along to give it to them.

AfroDite Superstar begins when AfroDite, a young inner-city woman (played by Simone Valentino, whose performance in this role won her the prize for best new star at the 2007 Feminist Porn Awards) is discovered at a karaoke club by Mr. Marcus, a hip-hop mogul who spots her star quality and decides to turn her into a great rap singer.

Now nothing can stop her, and with the help of her friend Isis (played by India), she makes records

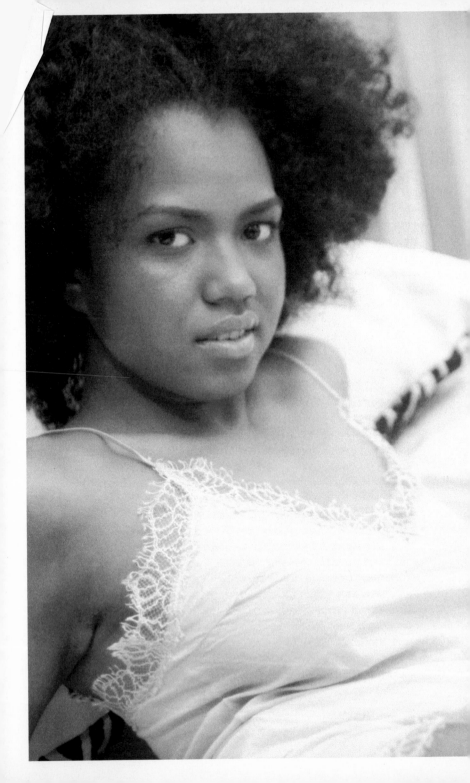

and videos, and she meets musicians, painters, and producers and has all kinds of sex with them, but it's always respectful, aesthetically pleasing, and accompanied by terrific music, which sets this sound track apart from the run-of-the-mill music typically featured in this kind of movie.

But her love for Mr. Marcus, who sees her only as a product that will make him rich, leaves her feeling unfulfilled, and even though he appears to redeem himself in the film's last scene, giving the story a happy ending (a trademark of the Royalle house), he still acts like a petty gangster on an ego trip, a type of man very common in the rap world.

As the opening credits roll, a fully clothed AfroDite is dancing to a hip-hop beat, with fairly clumsy moves that deepen the meaning of the scene and reinforce the healthy satirical message that Venus Hottentot wants to send as a way to show women of color in another light and offer a contrast to the way they're represented in pop culture and hip-hop videos—as sex objects whose only purpose is to shake their (always perfect) booties to the music.

Venus Hottentot actually doesn't define her films as porn. She views them as "intelligent mainstream work with explicit sexual content," along the lines of the work done by filmmakers like Larry Clark and John Cameron Mitchell.[11]

SEX MANNEQUIN
Director: Maria Beatty (France, 2007)

Maria Beatty, born in Caracas, Venezuela, and brought up in New York, now lives in Paris, where she runs Bleu Productions (www.bleuproductions .com). Beatty, who began producing and directing films more than fifteen years ago, before New Wave and alt porn were even conceived, is a pioneering figure in the new, artfully produced, beautifully

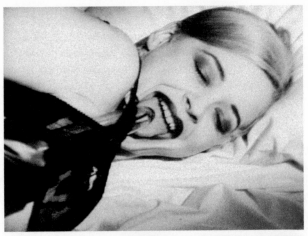

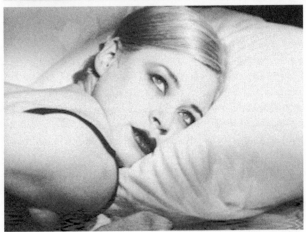

filmed adult movies focused on women's sexuality.

Beatty uses stories and fantasies that play out in fetishistic settings, and she's known for her in-depth explorations of female sexuality. Her artistic influences include German expressionist cinema, French surrealism, and American film noir, and her movies depict relationships between women that usually include BDSM, performed by actresses who have a modern, natural look.

Sex Mannequin is set in an abandoned loft

where a mannequin (played by London) comes to life to pleasure the main character (played by Dylan) with a full range of edgy lesbian sex games. We see incredibly spiky high heels, spanking, and bondage, and we hear plenty of moaning and dirty talk. In fact, that's precisely what is so sorely lacking in traditional porn—good, sexy dialogue that reveals the passion between the characters as they talk dirty to each other.

What I like about Maria Beatty's movies, and specifically about *Sex Mannequin*, is the way she uses such extreme close-ups of the performers' skin that you feel as if you can almost touch, smell, and taste the actresses. The sex scenes are staged like rituals, with the camera following the characters' desire so naturally that we almost come to believe that there's no camera at all, and that we're spying on a real couple.

OTHER NOTABLE FILMS BY MARIA BEATTY

1. *The Seven Deadly Sins* (2002)

2. *Lust* (2002)

3. *Ecstasy in Berlin, 1926* (2004)

4. *Silken Sleeves* (2006)

5. *Mask of Innocence* (2006)

6. *Coma* (2007)

7. *Boy in a Bathtub* (2007)

8. *Strap-On Motel* (2007)

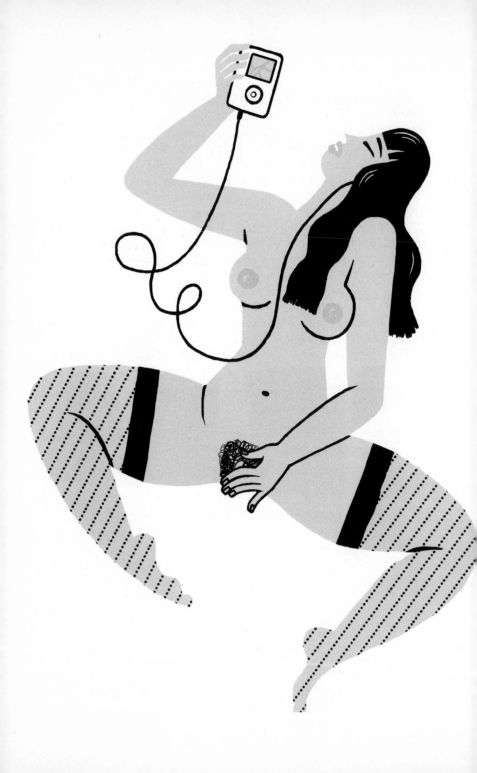

CHAPTER 10
RELAX AND ENJOY IT

In spite of all their peculiarities, adult movies are still just movies, and you can watch them however and wherever you please, guided only by your own comfort and convenience. You may like watching movies on the big screen, with popcorn and someone to talk with about the action. You may like watching in the comfort of your home, where the mighty remote lets you fast-forward through the dull parts and replay the highlights. Or maybe a plane flight is your time to catch up on the latest movies, thanks to eMule and a tiny iPod screen. You can do every one of these things with pornographic movies, too, even though you'll need a little more privacy because of porn's "side effects."

ALONE WITH AN ADULT MOVIE
As far as I'm concerned, you should watch porn wherever it most appeals to you—wherever it makes you hottest. Want a long relaxing session of solo sex, just you and your vibrator? Get comfortable on the living room couch or on your bed, light a few scented candles, and open a bottle of your favorite wine. Your pleasure will last as long as you want, and you certainly won't have to deal with anyone's failure to perform—but do make sure you have spare batteries on hand! If you run out, the party's over.

If you're traveling and find yourself alone and bored in a hotel room, your laptop is your best asset. You can pack your own erotic library, or if you have Internet access you can enjoy some streaming pornographic video. For another interesting use of your laptop, try IMing about a movie with your partner (if you're missing your partner) or maybe with some anonymous web surfer.

At work, if you're having a particularly stressful or boring day, close your office door and give orders that you're not to be disturbed, or escape to some discreet corner (maybe the restroom) with an iPod and a smartphone loaded with high-voltage goodies. That can send you back to work sporting a fresh perspective, and even looking a few years younger.

GIRLS' NIGHT

A little porn can also be a good way to liven up a night with the girls. If everybody's into it and nobody feels put off (this should be fun, so it's important for everyone to be comfortable), you can all watch a movie together and talk about how the long-haired guy turns you on (or how you wouldn't mind a little face time with the dark-haired leading lady), or about how you almost ended up in the hospital that time you tried the acrobatic position you're watching on the screen.

PARTNER PORN

There's also the possibility of partner porn, as long as your male partner is clear on the concept that watching porn with you is not a macho fest between himself and the film's male star, and that the point is not systematic duplication of sexual tableaux and stunts that are closer to contortionism than to what we normally understand as fucking. It should also be clear that the purpose of watching the movie is for both of you to get comfortable, get turned on, and have your own version of a spectacular screw. Finally, a word of caution—if you can't do without the popcorn, salt it lightly. You never know where your hands might end up during the movie—and salt stings!

TRAVELING COMPANIONS

When a guy watches porn, all he usually needs is his hand and a Kleenex. But we can get ourselves a trusty companion for our pleasure fests. And we're no longer limited to prosthetic-looking, nonsensuous plastic cocks—today we have our choice of many fabulous sex toys.

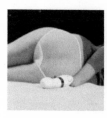 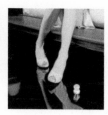 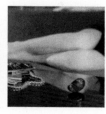 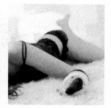

WHERE AND HOW SHOULD YOU WATCH PORN?

The following table presents the advantages and disadvantages of different possibilities for viewing adult films.

Where and How
On the couch
In a movie theater
In bed
With a partner
With women friends
On your iPod or smartphone

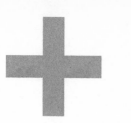

Pros	Cons
The couch is comfortable, relaxing, and close to the kitchen (for wine) and the bathroom (if you want a shower). And with the shades down and the curtains closed, it's very intimate.	If you don't make sure beforehand that none of your friends stop by, or that your mother won't be letting herself in to drop off a casserole, you could get so caught up in what you're doing that you won't realize what's happened until you hear a muffled scream and the sound of keys hitting the floor.
There aren't any theaters showing post-porn.* (Anyone want to organize a series?)	There's no intimacy at all, so this can only be a rehearsal of sorts. But you can buy the film later and watch it wherever you like.
I have nothing to say, pro or con—it's your bed!	I have nothing to say, pro or con—it's your bed!
You can have sex, laughs, hugs, tongue kisses, caresses, oral sex, "bite me there," "yes, yes," more hugs, "fuck me," and as much as you want—as if you yourself were the star of the porn film that the "other" actors are watching.	Your partner, especially a male partner, may think that everything he sees on the screen is to be taken seriously, and that it's your duty to turn yourself into his personal porn star.
You can make each other laugh, share an experience, and have a good time together.	One of you may be feeling put off by the movie without saying so.
Wherever you have your MP3 player or your smartphone, you have your own private viewing booth. And have you heard about the OhMiBod, the vibrator that connects to an iPod? Now, there's an advantage!	The iPod screen is very small, and if you look at it long enough, you'll end up with a wrinkle between your eyebrows from squinting to make out this or that butt or pair of nipples. And if you're watching on your phone, an urgent call midsession is a real turnoff.

* The term "post-porn," coined by the performance artist Annie Sprinkle, refers to the kind of independent, feminist porn described throughout this book.

Man
ife
sto

CHAPTER 11
ADULT FILMS FOR GROWN-UP WOMEN: A MANIFESTO

> *Women have arrived at last, and we're here to change porn.*

In the new adult films for grown-up women, I want to see women deciding how porn will represent us. I want to see women being women—women like you and me, women with feelings, education, and jobs, women who are mothers, married, divorced, and single, women who are lovers, young women and grown women, thin and curvy women, all enjoying their sexuality and enjoying themselves in the sexual situations that arise in movies.

The expression of women's sexuality is powerful, and maybe that bothers some men. Maybe they would rather believe that the only sexually attractive women are sluts, prostitutes, and hotties, and that all the rest are innocent creatures. Very few men like thinking about the sexuality of their mothers, sisters, and daughters. And yet the fact is, all of us are sexual beings, not just the Jenna Jamesons.

I don't plan to sit around waiting for a response from the pornographic film industry, and I'm not waiting around for the industry to reevaluate its fundamental, deeply rooted beliefs about female sexuality. If we don't do that ourselves, the industry certainly won't do it for us.

Our society has a tendency to dismiss porn as marginal and insignificant, to believe that it doesn't impinge on other areas of life. But it does. Porn isn't just porn. It's a discourse, a way of talking about sex. It's a way of seeing and understanding masculinity and femininity. But this discourse and the theory behind it are almost 100 percent male (and often sexist as well). There are almost no women's voices in this universe of discourse, just as there were no women's voices until recently in the worlds of politics and big business.

I believe that as women we have the right to enjoy adult films, and so I think we have to demand our share of the content of this discourse. We have to be creators—screenwriters, producers, and directors.

I recently became a mother, and when my daughter becomes a teenager and sees her first adult films, I think I'll want her to take away positive messages about sexuality, with feminist values and discourses. I don't want Rocco, Nacho, Marc Dorcel, Private, and Penthouse to be the ones explaining the world to her through sexually explicit films. It's not that I want to impose some kind of feminist censorship on the world of adult-oriented entertainment. The men who create that world will always have their point of view, and I accept and respect that. I just want their point of view not to be the only one. I want a porn with diversity of opinion.

Like it or not, these days we live in a porn-saturated society. There's porn all over the Internet,

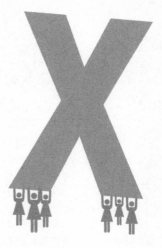

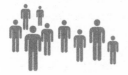

and there's porn in the media. Porn has come out of its dark closet. In this environment, it's very important for women to take a critical approach to porn, constantly analyzing and challenging the values that porn transmits.

The sexist values perpetuated by movies and advertising came in for a lot of criticism during the feminist explosion of the 1960s and 1970s. Women today need to bring the same critical awareness to adult films. We can't just turn our backs on porn and think it doesn't matter because men are the only ones looking at it. Even if that were true, what men are seeing and learning also affects us. Lots of men understand and interpret female sexuality through porn.

I believe that women's participation in pornographic discourse will give us an excellent opportunity to explain our sexuality to men in a way that's both vivid and explicit. What better way to help them grasp something that we know all about, but that they find so hard to understand?

TRANSLATOR'S NOTES

CHAPTER 1. PORN FOR MEN

1. Lucía Etxebarría, *Lo que los hombres no saben . . . el sexo contado por las mujeres* (Madrid: Casa del Libro, 2009). At this writing, there is no English-language edition.

CHAPTER 2. WOMEN, FEMINISM, AND PORNOGRAPHY

1. This passage was translated and adapted from the article "Machismo" as it appeared on the Wikipedia website when the Spanish edition went to press, and the passage is preserved in this edition for the sake of fidelity to the original volume. The Spanish term *machismo*, derived from *macho*, "male," is milder than English "misogyny" but stronger than "male chauvinism." For all practical purposes, the intensity of *machismo* and *macho* is roughly matched by that of English "sexism" and "sexist," two terms that are used in this translation in contexts where they sound more idiomatic in English.

2. The aphorism is actually "Pornography is the theory, and rape is the practice." It was formulated by Robin Morgan in her essay "Theory and Practice: Pornography and Rape," included in her collection *Going Too Far: The Personal Chronicle of a Feminist* (New York: Random House, 1977).

3. Wendy McElroy, *XXX: A Woman's Right to Pornography* (New York: St. Martin's, 1997).

4. Audacia Ray, "Feminist Porn Wars (New and Improved!) (Not Really)," blog at Waking Vixen Productions (www.waking vixen.com).

5. Lucía Etxebarría, *Lo que los hombres no saben . . . el sexo contado por las mujeres* (Madrid: Casa del Libro, 2009).

CHAPTER 3. THE HISTORY OF PORN

1. The Marquis Paul de Vibraye, who discovered an Upper Paleolithic representation of a woman around 1864 at Laugerie-Basse, in southwestern France, named the figurine *Vénus impudique* to distinguish his discovery from the "modest" Venuses of the Hellenistic style.

2. This misconception is widespread, no doubt because it seems so reasonable. But the word *fascinus* means "sorcery," "witchcraft," or "spell"—from the Latin infinitive *fascinare* ("to bewitch or enchant")—and is entirely without phallic connotations. In Roman times well before the eruption of Vesuvius, amulets bearing the image of an erect phallus were used as protective talismans. It was from this practice that a deity eventually evolved, one who retained his phallic image and was named Fascinus because of his existing association with protective spells.

3. In this translation, the word *mainstream,* unless used specifically in connection with pornography, indicates the broad cultural milieu in which, for example, first-run Hollywood films are released and reviewed. See chapter 5 for a definition of the phrase *mainstream porn.*

4. The FBI estimated that the film's actual earnings were much lower—around $100 million. Roger Ebert, in his review of *Inside Deep Throat* in the *Chicago Sun Times* (February 11, 2005), also estimated that the film's earnings were lower. *Deep Throat*, he wrote, "was made on the far fringes of the movie industry; [the film's director] later complained that most of the profits went to people he prudently refused to name as the mob. Since the mob owned most of the porn theaters in the pre-video days and inflated box office receipts as a way of laundering income from drugs and prostitution, it is likely, in fact, that *Deep Throat* did not really gross $600 million, although that might have been the box office tally." Michael Hiltzik added his voice to the discussion with two articles in the *Los Angeles Times*, "*Deep Throat* Numbers Just Don't Add Up" (February 24, 2005) and "Bad *Deep Throat* Numbers Are Multiplying" (March 10, 2005). The second of the two articles dismantled a

rebuttal to the first from Fenton Bailey and Randy Barbato, the writer and director of *Inside Deep Throat*. In the first article, Hiltzik not only disputed the $600 million figure (he called it "baloney") but also debunked claims that *Deep Throat* is the highest-grossing movie of all time: "The No. 1 mainstream movie of the 1970s . . . was *Star Wars*. To date, its domestic theatrical gross is $461 million. You want to tell me that *Deep Throat* has sold more tickets than *Star Wars*?" Regardless of its actual box office receipts, *Deep Throat* is probably the most financially successful *pornographic* film ever made.

5. Among many other actions against *Deep Throat*, two famous federal prosecutions of the film took place in the 1970s, one in Georgia (1975) and the other in Tennessee (1976).

CHAPTER 7. A WORD TO THE WISE WANKER

1. In the 1969 case of *Stanley v. Georgia*, the Supreme Court ruled that, with the exception of child pornography, private possession of pornography in the home was neither a crime nor subject to government regulation.

2. Jim Mitchell was convicted of voluntary manslaughter and served less than three years at San Quentin Prison. He was released in October 1997 and died of an apparent heart attack in July 2007.

3. Eric *Schaefer,* "Dirty Little Secrets: Scholars, Archivists, and Dirty Movies," *The Moving Image 5,* no. 2 (2005): 79–105.

4. Interview with Candida Royalle (www.candidaroyalle.com /faqs.txt).

5. The Panic Movement (*el Movimiento Pánico*) took its name from the god Pan and was centered on the three basic elements of terror, humor, and simultaneity. One aspect of the movement was Arrabal's well-known *teatro Pánico*, an absurdist, ritualistic approach to drama.

6. Eva Norvind drowned in Oaxaca, Mexico, in 2006.

7. In North American usage, the term *manga* generally refers to print cartoons, whereas *anime* denotes animated cartoons.

8. Most original video animations, or OVAs, are released in home video formats without first being screened in theaters

or shown on television. Some sources claim that *Cream Lemon*, released in August 1984, was not the first but the second *hentai* OVA, since the first episode of the *Lolita Anime* series of *hentai* OVAs had been released in February of that year.

9. Cited in "Our Story," at the Comstock Films website (www.comstockfilms.com/main.html).

10. See www.mortydiamond.com.

11. La Maleta Roja and Late Chocolate are adult boutiques based in Barcelona and Madrid, respectively, and the Late Late is a type of vibrator.

12. Linda Williams, *Screening Sex* (Chapel Hill, N.C.: Duke University Press, 2008). The passage cited here originally appeared as "Hard-Core Art Film: The Contemporary Realm of the Senses" in volume 13 of *Quadern portàtil*, a series published by the Museu d'Art Contemporani de Barcelona.

13. Beatriz Preciado (1970–) is a Spanish philosopher and queer theorist; André Bazin (1918-1958), an influential French film critic and film theorist, was cofounder of the French film journal *Cahiers du Cinéma*.

14. The phrase "politics of the gaze" derives from gaze theory, on which the American feminist critic Patricia Johnson has commented as follows: "'Looking' is not a simple, value-free activity. . . . Michel Foucault makes clear that the gaze is connected to power and surveillance: the person who gazes is empowered over the person who is the object of the gaze. A number of art and film critics have focused on the gender implications of this power imbalance, noting that implicit in the structures of much Western art and many classic Hollywood films is the idea of the male gazer and the female object. Within this context, Linda Nochlin in particular has addressed the issue, . . . arguing that the male artist's right to represent women is interconnected with the assumption of general male power over and control of women in society" (Patricia Johnson, "The Gendered Politics of the Gaze: Henry James and George Eliot," *Mosaic: A Journal for the Interdisciplinary Study of Literature* 30, no. 1 (1997): 39–54).

CHAPTER 8. SEXY SHOPPING

1. Chanelle Gallant, quoted by Tristan Taormino, "Political Smut Makers: Feminist Porn Takes Center Stage at Historic Event," *The Village Voice*, June 6, 2006.

CHAPTER 9. A SMORGASBORD OF ADULT FILMS

1. Nevertheless, we do know how the parties who own the rights to Fellini's film view Michael Lucas's remake. In February 2007 they sued Lucas Entertainment, Inc., and Lucas Distribution, Inc., for trademark and copyright infringement, but the judge at the preliminary injunction hearing refused to halt distribution of Lucas's film.

2. This is an allusion to "Paris vaut bien une messe," a probably apocryphal comment attributed to King Henry IV of France in connection with his decision to renounce Protestantism for Roman Catholicism and the French crown.

3. Linda Boreman later maintained that she never received a cent, and that the $1,250 payment went to Chuck Traynor, her husband at the time.

4. See chapter 3, note 4.

5. Boreman died in 2002 at the age of fifty-three from injuries sustained in a car crash. In the 1980s, she had become an antiporn activist.

6. Tristan Taormino, "Smart Ass Productions" (www.puckerup .com/smart_ass_video).

7. The alleged connection between *Debbie Does Dallas* and the State University of New York at Stony Brook has been reported as apocryphal in all likelihood and inconclusive at best. See Chris Mellides and Najib Aminy, "Debbie Did Not Do Stony Brook," *The Stony Brook Press*, July 20, 2008.

8. Marilyn Chambers died in April 2009, ten days short of her fifty-seventh birthday.

9. See chapter 7, note 2.

10. The film's publicity statement and a trailer for *Eastside Story* can be found at Vena Virago's website (wwwvena virago.com/movies.html).

11. See www.venushottentot.com.

CREDITS

Page 54 Emmanuelle © Alain Siritzky Productions; all others © VCA Pictures

Page 70 © Mistress Basia

Page 88 © Vivid Alt

Page 90 © RM Films International, www.russmeyer.com

Page 110 © Girls Gone Wild, www.girlsgonewild.com

Page 111 © (left) Girls Gone Wild, www.girlsgonewild.com; (middle and center) Internet Entertainment Group (IEG)

Page 121 © Mistress Basia

Page 128 © Loft Publications

Page 139 © Vivid Alt

Page 142 © Vivid Alt

Page 183 © Revolution Films

Page 185 © Andrew Blake

Page 186 © Andrew Blake

Page 190 © Innocent Pictures

Page 196 © FILMS A2

Page 198 © Evil Angel & enterbelladonna.com

Page 201 © ThinkFilm

Page 204 © Revolver Entertainment

Page 207 © Manga Films

Page 209 © Lust Films of Barcelona

Page 215 © Vivid Alt

Page 216 © Vivid Alt

Page 218 © Femme Productions

Page 220 © Maria Beatty

Page 225 © Lelo, www.lelo.com

Additional photography credits: Pablo Dobner, Guerrilla Girls, Richard In, Jalif, Anna Span, Erika Lust, Vanessa Glencross, Ovidie, José Rico, TheNotQuiteFool, Florent Gast, Pascal Lemoine, Chat Singh, VanessaGX, and loki777.

Illustrator Credits: Marion Dönneweg, Luci Gutierrez, Raimon Bragulat, Filip Zuan, Pau Santanach, Alberto Gabari, and Tassilo Rau.

ACKNOWLEDGMENTS

Thanks to Guillermo Hernáiz for talking to Editorial Melusina about me (and saying such nice things); to José Pons and Ana S. Pareja at Melusina for their faith in this project and their help in making it a reality; to Marion Dönneweg for bringing her artistic talents to bear on this book's design while awaiting the birth of her son Felix; to Pablo Dobner for his collaboration on almost every aspect of this book; to Monica Escudero for all her great help with research and editing; and to my daughter Lara for giving me time, during the first year of her life, to give birth to this book.

ABOUT THE AUTHOR

Erika Lust (Stockholm, Sweden, 1977) is a filmmaker, journalist, and cofounder of Lust Films. She is the director of two award-winning adult films: *Five Hot Stories for Her* (2007), which won Best Movie of the Year at the Feminist Porn Awards in Toronto and *Barcelona Sex Project* (2008), an experimental independent documentary, which won Best Erotic Documentary at the E-Line Awards in Berlin. Her most recent film is called *Life, Love & Lust* (2010). Lust lives in Barcelona.

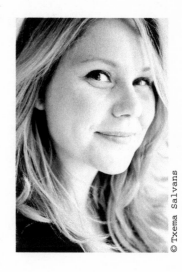

© Txema Salvans

SELECTED TITLES FROM SEAL PRESS

For more than thirty years, Seal Press has published groundbreaking books. By women. For women. Visit our website at www.sealpress.com. Check out the Seal Press blog at www.sealpress.com/blog.

Dirty Girls: Erotica for Women, edited by Rachel Kramer Bussel. $15.95, 978-1-58005-251-1. A collection of tantalizing and steamy stories compiled by prolific erotica writer Rachel Kramer Bussel.

Sexier Sex: Lessons from the Brave New Sexual Frontier, by Regina Lynn. $14.95, 978-1-58005-231-3. A fun, provocative guide to discovering your sexuality and getting more pleasure from your sensual life.

Sexual Intimacy for Women: A Guide for Same-Sex Couples, by Glenda Corwin, Ph.D. $16.95, 978-1-58005-303-7. In this prescriptive and poignant book, Glenda Corwin, PhD, helps female couples overcome obstacles to sexual intimacy through her examination of the emotional, physical, and psychological aspects of same-sex relationships.

Getting Off: A Woman's Guide to Masturbation, by Jamye Waxman, illustrations by Molly Crabapple. $15.95, 978-1-58005-219-1. Empowering and female-positive, this is a comprehensive guide for women on the history and mechanics of the oldest and most common sexual practice.

Sex and Bacon: Why I Love Things That Are Very, Very Bad for Me, by Sarah Katherine Lewis. $14.95, 978-1-58005-228-3. A sensual— and sometimes raunchy—book celebrating the intersection of sex and food.

Fucking Daphne: Mostly True Stories and Fictions, edited by Daphne Gottlieb. $15.95, 978-1-58005-235-1. An erotic collection of stories—all centered on the fictional character "Daphne"—that blurs the line between fact and fantasy.